Training for Community Health

T0177572

Training for Community Health

Bridging the Global Healthcare Gap

Edited by

Anne Geniets

James O'Donovan

Laura Hakimi

Niall Winters

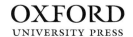

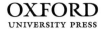

OXFORD
UNIVERSITY PRESS

Great Clarendon Street, Oxford, OX2 6DP,
United Kingdom

Oxford University Press is a department of the University of Oxford.
It furthers the University's objective of excellence in research, scholarship,
and education by publishing worldwide. Oxford is a registered trade mark of
Oxford University Press in the UK and in certain other countries

First Edition published in 2021

Impression: 1

Published in the United States of America by Oxford University Press
198 Madison Avenue, New York, NY 10016, United States of America

British Library Cataloguing in Publication Data

Data available

Library of Congress Control Number: 2020952971

ISBN 978–0–19–886624–4

DOI: 10.1093/oso/9780198866244.001.0001

Printed and bound by
CPI Group (UK) Ltd, Croydon, CR0 4YY

To all the community health workers—for your tireless efforts to bridge the global healthcare gap.

Anne Geniets

To my parents—thank you for always supporting me.
To my Village Health Team colleagues and friends of Seeta Nazigo Parish, Uganda—thank you for teaching me and for your service. Webale nyo.

To my wife Stephanie—thank you for everything.

James O'Donovan

To my Dad. RIP.

Niall Winters

Foreword

Sonia E. Sachs and Jeffrey D. Sachs

This rich compendium of research for methods on enhancing the education, training, and supervision of community health workers (CHWs) comes at a crucial time. The global relevance of well-trained, well-managed, and professionalized CHWs remains as urgent as ever. CHWs are the front-line workers to help communities to stay safe, to seek medical health when ill, to watch for symptoms among the population, and to create the trust between policymakers and the citizenry. The Covid-19 epidemic is not the first emerging disease of our time and it won't be the last, alas. CHWs will be more essential than ever in the years ahead to fight such epidemics and to support health systems generally.

Both extensive experience and scholarly studies demonstrate that a network of local, trained, supervised, and remunerated personnel with responsibility for the wellbeing of 100–200 households in their own community can be enormously beneficial for maintaining the community's health and for preventing premature deaths of mothers and children. Additionally, this cadre is uniquely positioned, indeed irreplaceable, for real-time surveillance of incidence of diseases in the community, especially infectious diseases like HIV, Ebola, Zika, or Covid-19. Working in their own home community, CHWs become aware of new diseases or of the increasing frequency of existing diseases at their early manifestation and are therefore vital to alert public health professionals immediately, with the potential to contain an early outbreak before it becomes a major epidemic.

In the case of an epidemic, it is the CHWs who are best positioned to help contain and suppress the disease. The comparative advantage of these local health workers is that they know the community and in return, the community knows and trusts them. The public is disposed to heed their advice, much more so than the advice of an outsider, who often faces intense distrust. Indeed, the vital importance of such trust is the case whether the setting is a low-income or high-income country. As a pertinent example, a group of highly respected health professionals have called for a 'National UK program of community health workers for Covid-19 response' (Haines et al., 2020).

Despite the enormous benefits of the CHW cadre, CHWs are rarely formalized as part of public health strategy. Accepting CHWs as a formal, indeed vital, human resource for public health has a long and tortuous history, with fits and starts in many countries but almost no cases where CHWs have become a formal, trained, supervised, and remunerated cadre within a national public health system. Indeed, in rich countries, CHWs have rarely been deployed, because of an erroneous perception that public health can be delivered adequately by doctors and nurses. Such a deep misunderstanding is certainly widespread in the USA. In low- and middle-income countries with woefully inadequate health budgets, CHWs are typically community-based volunteers who themselves are poor and so cannot be held accountable for working consistently because of the need to pursue their own livelihoods, such as tending to their small farms. Most CHW initiatives in such settings are therefore patchy and small-scale efforts of non-governmental organizations, frequently one-off, short-term, narrowly focused, and basically disconnected from the rest of the health system. Governments in very low-income countries cannot afford at this point to set up national-scale, formal, professionalized, and remunerated CHWs as part of the national healthcare strategy, even though CHWs would have enormous social and health benefits at remarkably low cost. And unfortunately most donor agencies have overlooked the importance of CHWs in their own donor financing for the health sector.

CHWs and Universal Health Coverage

In the era of Sustainable Development Goals (SDGs), and notably the call for Universal Health Coverage as part of SDG 3, there has been an increase of rhetorical support for CHWs but little more actual donor commitment or government investment in them. Nonetheless, CHWs are a *sine qua non* for Universal Health Coverage for two main reasons. In low-income settings such as in sub-Saharan Africa, there are insufficient numbers of doctors and nurses, especially in rural areas. The education and salaries of doctors and nurses at the scale required has until today been an unmanageable burden on the country's health budget. And ironically, after the government invests in the long and expensive education of nurses and doctors, these well-trained professionals, understandably, emigrate and contribute to the health workforce of richer countries, often lured deliberately by those richer countries. CHWs, on the other hand, are volunteers or have much lower salaries, can be trained and deployed within a short amount of time, and are not lured by richer countries. For a secondary-school graduate in a poor farming community, becoming a CHW is an excellent career path, perhaps one that will ultimately lead to becoming a trained nurse, and in any event offers skills training and a rewarding vocation sometimes at a salary well above the poverty line. If all of sub-Saharan Africa were to deploy CHW cadres at the needed scale, around two million good jobs would be created.

In low-income rural settings, large numbers of women and children die of a handful of conditions that are preventable or treatable by interventions that CHWs can deploy. These include communicable diseases such as malaria, nutrition-related diseases that can be addressed through dietary supplementation, and pregnancy and parturition-related causes. When trained to deal with this handful of clinical entities, and some easily managed noncommunicable disorders, CHWs can significantly reduce mortality rates, especially when integrated into properly designed systems of CHWs with supervisors, emergency transport, clinical facilities, and data systems.

CHWs are also highly effective because they develop long-term relationships with families, so that they know the family's physical and social surroundings, the composition of the household, and issues related to the family's access to food, medicines, clinic follow-up, and difficulties of complying with the doctor's advice and prescriptions. In the absence of a CHW, a patient's health can deteriorate so much that by the time the patient arrives at the clinic, the disease process has advanced too far to redress. For this reason capitated insurance companies in rich countries are starting to cover the costs of community outreach personnel who reduce the frequency of re-admissions to hospitals by helping patients adhere to the outpatient regime.

Technological innovations have dramatically enlarged the scope of the CHW's life-saving interventions. The advent of long-lasting insecticide treated bed nets to fight malaria, combined with highly effective artemisinin-based treatments and rapid diagnostic tests, have made the CHWs the leaders of the highly successful efforts over the past 15 years to cut the deaths from malaria in rural Africa. There are now many other point-of-service rapid diagnostic technologies that can be deployed, such as blood pressure checks, pulse oximeter for oxygen saturation, blood sugar testing, and pregnancy testing. CHWs have also been routinely dispensing many treatments in the household under supervision and consultation with a supervisor. Common examples include oral rehydration solution and zinc for uncomplicated diarrhoea, ready-to-use therapeutic food for some cases of severe acute malnutrition, and antibiotics for uncomplicated pneumonia.

Perhaps the greatest recent transformation in healthcare in low-income settings has been the advent of new Information and Communication Technologies (ICTs). The use of smartphones and tablets in systems delivery in poor rural communities has been a game-changer. The almost ubiquitous mobile phone coverage in sub-Saharan Africa, and the rapidly declining costs of mobile phones and tablets, have made it possible to empower CHWs with these enormously useful technologies. There is the obvious use of the phones for consultations with supervisors, including getting supportive supervision, and the rising use of phones for telemedicine consultations and emergency referrals. Additionally, and perhaps less obviously, the smartphone provides easy-to-use point-of-service job aids, visuals for counselling, reminders for follow-up, algorithms for decision support, and the unprecedented advantages of gathering and using real-time data garnered during a household visit.

Indeed the unprecedented and transformative benefit of digital health is the availability and use of real-time data for ongoing feedback loops, allowing continuous adaptive implementation and quality improvement of healthcare services, including personalized feedback to CHWs. There is automatically generated information such as GPS and useful data that is collected as the CHW routinely uses the phone to register family members, and to record test results, diagnoses, and treatments provided. The CHW and the supervisor can then review the data together at the end of the week to see what information can be gleamed about the community's health, looking for new epidemic outbreaks or evidence of failures of the health system, and discussing how well a CHW dealt with issues as they arose. Together the CHW and supervisor can review the CHW working conditions and engage in continuous supportive supervision with the aim of targeted, skill-specific re-training and other management decisions based, in part, on automatically generated data. Managers can track the number and time of household visits by the CHW and adjust the ratio of clients to providers. They can track use of commodities, cross-linking them with tests administered and treatments provided, being able to adjust the supply chain, track productivity and quality of care and provide ongoing specific re-training, education, and mutual performance evaluation in support of overall health system accountability.

Our Experience in the Millennium Villages

Our own experience with professionalized CHWs comes from a ten-year demonstration project we carried out during 2005–2015 known as the Millennium Villages Project (MVP) (Mitchell et al., 2018). The MVP consisted of clusters of remote rural communities within ten countries of sub-Saharan Africa where we collaborated with the communities to demonstrate the feasibility of community's deployment of systems to improve food production, access to education, health, infrastructure, and business development.

The basic unit of the MVP health system provided continuum of care for about 5000 villagers. Every household had a designated CHW who was responsible for a panel of 100–150 households, depending on density of distribution of dwellings, topography of the terrain, and the disease burden. A clinic for the 5000 people living within walkable distance, was upgraded to have the capacity to do prevention and treatment of basic maternal and child health; to have the capability for safe childbirth with 24/7 basic emergency obstetric care and emergency transportation to a local rural hospital for comprehensive emergency obstetric care. In 2008, mobile phones used by CHWs were upgraded to smartphones with CommCare, an application co-formulated with Dimagi, which supported the decision-making of the CHWs on the daily rounds of their panel of households. CommCare application provided support structure for longitudinal care of all children under five and women of reproductive age, focusing in detail on all the main milestones of especially the first thousand days, starting from conception to the age of two, making sure that all necessary interventions, like vaccination, took place, and on time (CommCare, 2020).

We set up a Millennium Village Information System which was a web-based, multi-sectoral, real-time, and near real-time monitoring system of data. The daily real-time data from CHWs, from hub-based monthly data from clinics and schools, quarterly data from agro-business, and annual data from rapid infrastructure and facility assessment, together constituted an integrated MV information system. The continuous integrated data allowed for timely feedback loops that improved oversight of service delivery and of status of infrastructure, equipment, supply chain, training, and supervision. The village team and village committees used the information system to monitor and evaluate the programme of each sector (agriculture, infrastructure, health, education, and business development), using the feedback loops for ongoing adaptive implementation of interventions and of management systems, with continuous quality improvement.

We reconstructed a tool called Verbal Autopsy, previously used only in research, to become an operational tool that would regularly examine failures and gaps in the health system delivery. Interviews sensitively carried out with next of kin were conducted by a CHW on a smartphone application soon after the vital event. Subsequently, using an automated algorithm—to obviate the need for high-level clinicians to make the diagnosis—the team had information on the approximate cause deaths of all women and children in the community. We designed a complementary tool that we called Social Autopsy which was also a smartphone application asking questions that helped, by using an algorithm, to identify the proximate cause of the 'three delays', or obstacles, to getting possible life-saving care. The health team reviewed the automatically generated monthly reports of the Verbal and Social Autopsies and were able to address in near real-time the revealed gaps in the health delivery system. The health team—CHWs, CHW supervisors, nurses, managers, and village leadership—held frequent 'morbidity and mortality rounds' to learn from these findings and discuss solutions. This participatory exercise done with community representatives, CHWs, and the local health team was part of a collaborative effort where everyone, including the families themselves had a role, and a responsibility, to continuously and regularly refine the healthcare delivery system in order to keep improving the health of the community.

SDG 3, Covid-19, and the Way Forward

The Covid-19 pandemic is not only a profound global tragedy and disaster; it is also an urgent wake-up call to the need for effective public health systems in all countries. In this pandemic, many rich countries, including the USA, have performed badly—one can say miserably—because of the failure to launch a public health response to the epidemic, including testing, contact tracing, and helping infected individuals to self-isolate at home or quarantine in public facilities. Countries such as Cambodia, Lao PDR, and Vietnam, by contrast, were able to suppress the epidemic quickly and effectively through the deployment of public health cadres. If only the USA and hard-hit Western European countries had had a cadre of CHWs to help implement the needed public health response.

Perhaps this time the USA will learn from the disaster of Covid-19, just as the East Asian countries learned to build public health systems after the outbreak of SARS in 2003 and H1N1 in 2009–2010. In fact, fully 73 years after health was declared to be a basic human right in the Universal Declaration of Human Rights and the constitution of the World Health Organization, both in 1948, and 43 years after the Alma-Alta Declaration in 1978 that called for 'Health for All by the Year 2000,' perhaps the whole world will finally achieve what we have repeatedly promised all these decades: universal health coverage for every person on the planet. Notably, the 72nd World Health Assembly in May 2019 passed a resolution recognizing the vital importance of CHWs for achieving Universal Health Coverage and calling on all member states to implement the newly produced WHO guidelines on CHWs.

The Covid-19 disaster shows us the urgent need for universal health coverage. The successes of public health systems supported by CHWs and the digital technologies, show us the way forward. The SDG 3 gives us a shared global timeline to 2030 to fulfil this goal. This important volume of studies is therefore exactly what is needed: a guide and roadmap to success, providing invaluable guidance to health system leaders, policymakers, and local staff, to bring about the revolution in healthcare that can save millions of lives per year and protect us from the dire threats of newly emerging diseases. When SDG 3 is finally achieved, and it will be, the CHWs will surely have played an indispensable role, supported by the wise counsel in the articles in this volume.

References

CommCare (2020). CommCare—the world's most powerful mobile data collection platform. Available from: https://www.dimagi.com/commcare/

Haines, A., Falceto de Barros, E., Berlin, A., Heymann, D., & Harris, M. (2020). National UK programme of community health workers for Covid-19 response. *Lancet*, 395(10231), 1173–1175.

Mitchell, S., Gelman, A., Ross, R., Chen, J., Bari, S., Huynh, K.U., et al. (2018). The Millennium Villages Project: A retrospective, observational, end-line evaluation. *Lancet Global Health*, 6(5), E500–E513.

Contents

Abbreviations

3ie	International Initiative for Impact Evaluation
ABCD	acquire, bond, comprehend, and defend
AC	agent communautaire
ACT	artemisinin-based combination therapy
ADR	action design research
AHW	auxiliary health workers
ANC	antenatal care
ANM	auxiliary nurse midwives
APE	agentes polivalentes elementare
ASCSD	Accelerated Strategy of Child Survival and Development
ASHA	accredited social health activist
CDVC	care delivery value chain
CHEW	community health extension workers
CHT	community health toolkit
CHV	community health volunteers
CHW	community health worker
CLSP	community-level service provider
COPE	community outreach and patient empowerment
CoPs	communities of practice
CU	community unit
DIV	Development Innovation Programme
DOT	directly observed therapy
DPME	Department of Planning, Monitoring and Evaluation
DRC	Democratic Republic of Congo
eCDA	electronic clinical decision algorithms
EIDM	evidence-informed decision-making
EU	European Union
FCHV	female community health volunteers
FMOH	Federal Ministry of Health in Ethiopia
GDPR	General Data Protection Regulation
GPG	global public good
HAD	health development army
HCD	human-centred design
HELP	health enablement and learning platform
HEW	health extension workers
HSLD	health systems leadership development
iCCM	integrated community case management
ICT	information and communication technologies
IHME	Institute for Health Metrics and Evaluation

IMCI	integrated management of childhood illness
IMPaCT	individualized management for patient-centred targets
ISO	International Standards Organization
IVR	interactive-voice response
KTU	knowledge transfer unit
LMH	Last Mile Health
LMIC	low and middle-income country
MDAT	Malawi Development Assessment Tool
MESH-QI	mentorship and enhanced supervision for healthcare and quality improvement
mHealth	mobile health
MNCH	maternal, neonatal, and child health
MoHP	Ministry of Health and Population
MOOC	massive open access online course
MVP	Millennium Villages Project
NCD	non-communicable diseases
NDHS	Nepal Demographic and Health Survey
NGO	non-governmental organization
ODK	open data kit
ORS	oral rehydration salts
ORT	oral rehydration therapy
PEPFAR	The President's Emergency Plan for AIDS Relief
PHC	primary healthcare
PIH	Partners in Health
QES	qualitative evidence synthesis
RCT	randomized controlled trial
RDT	rapid diagnostic test
RUTF	ready-to-use therapeutic foods
SDG	sustainable development goal
STS	science and technology studies
TBA	traditional birth attendant
TEL	technology-enhanced learning
UHC	Universal Health Care
UN	United Nations
WDG	women's development group
WHO	World Health Organization

Contributors

Ṣẹ̀yẹ Abímbọ́lá
Senior Lecturer and Research Fellow
School of Public Health
University of Sydney
Sydney, New South Wales, Australia

Michael Bailey
Director Digital Solutions
Community Health Academy
Last Mile Health
Baltimore, MD, USA

Julia Berman
Chief Partnerships Officer
Muso
San Francisco, CA, USA

Celia Brown
Associate Professor
Division of Health Sciences
University of Warwick
Coventry, Warwickshire, UK

Magnus Conteh
Executive Director
Community Health Academy
Last Mile Health
Baltimore, MD, USA

Nigel Fancourt
Associate Professor
Department of Education
University of Oxford
Oxford, UK

Karen Finnegan
Associate Scientific Director, Pivot
Department of Global Health and Social
Medicine
Harvard Medical School
Boston, MA, USA

Sanjay Gadi
Medical Student
Harvard Medical School
Harvard University
Boston, MA, USA

Anne Geniets
Post-Doctoral Research Fellow
Department of Education
University of Oxford
Oxford, UK

Laura Hakimi
Post-Doctoral Research Fellow
Department of Education
University of Oxford
Oxford, UK

Jade Vu Henry
Visiting Post-Doctoral Researcher
Department of Sociology
Goldsmiths, University of London
London, UK

Isaac Holeman
Chief Research Officer, Medic, and Clinical
Assistant Professor
Department of Global Health
University of Washington
Seattle, WA, USA

Maureen Kelley
Professor of Bioethics
Ethox Centre, Nuffield Department of
Population Health
University of Oxford
Oxford, UK

Alice S. Lakati
Dean
School of Public Health
Amref International University
Nairobi, Kenya

Laurenz Langer
Senior Researcher
Africa Centre for Evidence
University of Johannesburg
Johannesburg, Gauteng, South Africa

Lesley-Anne Long
Senior Advisor to the Executive Director
Community Health Academy
Last Mile Health
Baltimore, MD, USA

David Musoke
Lecturer
Disease Control and Environmental Health
Makerere University School of Public Health
Kampala, Uganda

Shobhana Nagraj
MRC Clinical Research Training Fellow
Nuffield Department of Women's &
Reproductive Health
University of Oxford
Oxford, UK

Promise Nduku
Researcher
Africa Centre for Evidence
University of Johannesburg
Johannesburg, South Africa

James O'Donovan
Director of Research
Division of Research and Health Equity
Omni Med Uganda
Makata, Uganda

Peter Otieno
Operations Lead
Amref Health Africa
Nairobi, Kenya

Daniel Palazuelos
Assistant Professor
BWH Division of Global Health Equity
Harvard Medical School
Boston, MA, USA

Raj Panjabi
U.S. Global Malaria Coordinator for the
President's Malaria Initiative
Harvard Medical School
Boston, MA, USA

Moshidi Putuka
Junior Researcher
Africa Centre for Evidence
University of Johannesburg
Johannesburg, Gauteng, South Africa

Zafeer Ravat
Researcher
Africa Centre for Evidence
University of Johannesburg
Johannesburg, Gauteng, South Africa

Jeffrey D. Sachs
University Professor and Director of the
Center for Sustainable Development
Earth Institute
Columbia University
New York, USA

Sonia E. Sachs
Research Scholar
Center for Sustainable Development
Earth Institute
Columbia University
New York, USA

Nkululeko Tshabalala
Researcher
Africa Centre for Evidence
University of Johannesburg
Johannesburg, South Africa

Beatrice Wasunna
Senior Researcher
Department of Research and Learning
Medic
Nairobi, Kenya

Niall Winters
Professor of Education and Technology
Department of Education
University of Oxford
Oxford, UK

1
Introduction

Anne Geniets, James O'Donovan, Laura Hakimi, and Niall Winters

The Health Equity Gap

Over a decade ago, the World Health Organization (WHO) identified a severe shortage of healthcare workers in the global health workforce (WHO, 2006), with rural and low-income settings being disproportionately affected (Global Health Workforce Alliance, 2013). Simultaneously, emerging evidence suggested that the deployment of community health workers (CHWs) in these areas was helping to increase access to basic healthcare, particularly for underserved population groups (Lehmann & Sanders, 2007). More than a decade later, as highlighted in particular by the Ebola outbreak in West Africa and the worldwide Covid-19 pandemic, CHWs have become an essential part of an increasingly stretched, yet interconnected, global health workforce. In many ways, the Covid-19 pandemic laid bare the stark health equity gaps between the poorest and most vulnerable and those who can afford access to healthcare, not just in low resource settings, but all around the world. Ultimately, the role of CHWs is to bridge this gap, and in doing so strengthen health systems by connecting and triaging those with limited or no access to formal healthcare services. To respond effectively to the ever-changing needs of local communities, resource- and staff-shortages, and to new public health challenges requires a flexible and adaptable CHW workforce.

Training and supervision have been cited as integral aspects of well-functioning CHW programmes (WHO, 2018). However, to date little research has focused on addressing this specific topic, and so we have brought together world-leading practitioners and academics, from different geographic regions, to contribute to this edited volume. The aim of the book is to provide researchers, practitioners, and graduate students with a comprehensive and multifaceted overview of CHW training and supervision, and position it as a core area of global health. The book builds on theoretical and methodological research, drawing in particular on studies of health worker practice, to better understand ways of designing effective and adaptable CHW training and supervision programmes.

Anne Geniets, James O'Donovan, Laura Hakimi, and Niall Winters, *Introduction* In: *Training for Community Health*. Edited by: Anne Geniets, James O'Donovan, Laura Hakimi, and Niall Winters, Oxford University Press. © Oxford University Press 2021. DOI: 10.1093/oso/9780198866244.003.0001

The Multifaceted Roles of CHWs

The deployment of CHWs to increase access to Primary Health Care (PHC) services is not new. In the late 1800s, in Eastern Europe and in Russia, lay health workers, known as 'feldshers', were trained and deployed as paramedics to provide emergency care services (Sidel, 1968). In the 1930s, partially influenced by the feldshers' success, China introduced so-called 'Farmer Scholars'. In this project, illiterate farmers in rural areas of China were trained to 'record births and deaths, vaccinate against smallpox and other diseases, give first aid and health education talks, and help communities keep their wells clean' (Rifkin, 2017, p. 93). The Farmer Scholars were the predecessors of China's barefoot doctor programme, of which there were almost one million at the programme's height in 1972, serving an estimated population of 800 million people (Rosenthal & Greiner, 1982). It was the success of the barefoot doctors' model, which was developed as part of China's infamous Cultural Revolution (Mathers & Huang, 2014), that inspired the establishment of many CHW programmes in other parts of the world, including India, Tanzania, and Venezuela.

In the 1960s and 1970s, with many countries failing to address the health needs of underserved groups of society through traditional hospital-based models of care, the need for alternative, community-based models of healthcare delivery became increasingly apparent. Today's CHW programmes can mostly be traced back to the Alma-Ata Declaration of 1978, which was adopted at the International Conference on Primary Health Care and established health as a human right. To guarantee this right to health, the declaration tasked governments with the responsibility of designing policies, strategies, and programmes that deliver healthcare closer to where people live and work. It articulated a vision of primary health that relied on teams of providers at the local level. These providers would include: 'physicians, nurses, midwives, auxiliaries and community workers as applicable, as well as traditional practitioners as needed, suitably trained socially and technically to work as a health team and to respond to the expressed health needs of the community' (WHO, 1978, p. 2). Over the following decade, community workers and traditional practitioners were recruited into CHW programmes which came to be regarded as a cornerstone for an integrated primary care system (Global Health Work Force Alliance, 2010).

Yet, despite many countries rolling out CHW-led PHC programmes, a culmination of factors in the 1980s and 1990s led to the demise of many such initiatives. Programmes were disjointed, lacked funding, and were seen by some governments as 'second-class' models of care delivery. In addition, the global oil crisis of the 1970s resulted in a debt crisis which affected many low and middle-income countries (LMICs) in the 1980s. Governments were forced to embrace free market reforms by many international donors, and to reduce public sector financing. This caused a decrease in overall government spend on primary care and resulted in many CHW programmes falling by the wayside (Perry, 2013; Perry et al., 2014).

However, by the early to mid-2000s, a renewed interest in CHW programmes was evident. Indeed, over the past decade, CHWs have received significant attention due to their potential in helping to address the global shortage of trained professional health workers, while at the same time increasing care delivery to underserved populations (Oliver et al., 2015). In the context and aftermath of the Covid-19 pandemic, and with a global shortage of 7.2 million healthcare professionals (a number that is projected to rise to 13 million in the next 15 years (WHO, 2013)), this interest is set to intensify over the decades to come.

To date, however, CHWs' roles, power, levels of training, supervision, and renumeration continue to vary widely. This diversity is also reflected in the nearly 70 terms used to describe and characterize CHWs, ranging from 'activista' to 'barefoot doctors' (Ballard et al., 2018). It has become evident that the role and tasks of CHWs need to be viewed both in relation to the health systems within which they operate and to other healthcare professionals (Olaniran et al., 2017). In light of this diversity, and accounting for the variety of different CHW groups, defining the professional requirements of CHWs has become a priority: without a clear definition of these tasks and roles, the adaptation of policies to fast-changing environments becomes difficult. Having a flexible and adaptable CHW workforce, which can be trained in new skills and rapidly deployed, is critical, but to fulfil this role successfully, they require regular training and supervision (WHO, 2007).

The Role of Training and Supervision for CHWs

Among the many challenges facing CHWs—each one being important in its own right—this book will specifically address the issue of *CHW training and supervision*. For the purpose of this book, training refers to the *initial* process of skill acquisition and teaching; supervision refers to the process of *on-going support*, thereby 'helping staff to improve their own work performance continuously... with a focus on using supervisory visits as an opportunity to improve knowledge and skills' (O'Donovan et al., 2018). In subsequent chapters of this edited volume, contributors discuss the diverse array of models of CHW training and supervision—from in-person training, to remote supervision supported by mobile technologies—and the challenges of designing and implementing these approaches successfully.

Indeed, the contextual challenges around CHW training and supervision are numerous. They include, for example: infrastructural and logistical challenges (such as gathering CHWs together in the same place for regular training sessions), a lack of funding for training and supervision sessions, and competing professional and personal interests, especially in those countries where CHWs work on a voluntary basis (Ludwick et al., 2018; Scott et al., 2018). Moreover, these obstacles are compounded by an ever-increasing number of tasks expected of CHWs, which can result in feelings of exhaustion and disempowerment among CHWs (O'Donovan et al., 2020).

Amidst the tension of these competing interests, training CHWs as 'reflective prac-titioners', who engage in social learning and remain adaptive to the ever-changing needs of their local communities and to the latest advances in healthcare, requires in-novative thinking. Alternative approaches to programme design are thus needed: ap-proaches that conceptualize CHW training and supervision as the *practice* of social learning. In other words, to achieve continuous, structured, up-to-date training and supervision, it is necessary to start with a strong *pedagogy*, that is, the method and practice of teaching. The question then becomes, what pedagogy to use? Given CHWs' role in working with the most underserved to bridge the health equity gap, it is evident that a suitable pedagogy requires a strong social justice perspective, and that it be an *equitable* pedagogy—one that recognizes that knowledge is power. *Critical pedagogy* answers this call. It is not only a way to equip a skilled, adaptable, equitable, and reflective healthcare workforce, but to address the many medical challenges still facing under-resourced populations in the 21st century.

As Paulo Freire has argued in *A Pedagogy of the Oppressed*, critical pedagogy con-ceptualizes education as a practice of freedom (Freire, 1970). In this equitable defin-ition of pedagogy, experience can be regarded a valid form of knowledge, and learning is understood as a continuing process of 'participation' rather than a discrete instance of knowledge 'acquisition' (Sfard, 1998). An equitable pedagogy therefore seeks to combine the understanding of participation as learning with training for evidence-based interventions, incorporating reflection, evaluations, and monitoring as essen-tial components. This approach thus encourages a relational engagement with—and between—CHWs, rather than a top-down pedagogy that reinforces current power imbalances. Accordingly, a greater emphasis on the pedagogy of CHW programmes prioritizes high quality and high impact training over fast scaling up of projects (Winters et al., 2018a).

While multiple views prevail on what it means to learn, and on how learning leads to social change (ranging from behaviourist to constructivist and cognitivist ap-proaches) (Ertmer & Newby, 2013), social theories of learning recognize the import-ance of the context (e.g. the educational environment) and the community in which learning occurs (e.g. communities of practice) (Bahn, 2001). Importantly, we sug-gest that this social conceptualization of learning is particularly important for CHW training and supervision. As time is a key aspect of social learning, we further em-phasize the importance of ongoing training and supervision, which, unfortunately, has typically been the most neglected phase of training (O'Donovan et al., 2018), with significant variability in terms of how it is delivered (Redick et al., 2014).

The training picture becomes even more complicated when challenges in defining educational objectives and outcomes are considered. Questions such as, 'How can learning be evaluated? How can long-term retention be assessed? Does training bring about desired change in practice and how can this be captured and evaluated?' have often been posed by academics and practitioners alike and still occupy those working in the field of CHW training and supervision (Ruiz et al., 2012; Winters et al., 2017). When set against differing cultural interpretations and expectations of what it means to be trained and supervised, this only adds to the complexity of the topic at hand. For example, what it means to be trained and supervised as a CHW in Kenya is likely to be very different to a CHW in the USA. Indeed, there can be drastic in-country variations in expectations, yet these socially-nuanced and complex aspects of CHW training and supervision have often been overlooked in the existing literature (Altobelli, 2017).

Contextual Aspects: Digital Health Interventions and the Role of Technology

mHealth can be broadly defined as 'mobile computing, medical sensor, and communications technologies for healthcare' (O'Donovan et al., 2015). As outlined in a seminal paper published by Labrique and team in 2013, mobile technologies have several roles in assisting health systems strengthening, one of which is to support the education and training of health professionals (Labrique et al., 2013). mHealth has been suggested to be particularly important in LMIC settings, given the high ownership of mobile phones, especially in the context of sub-Saharan Africa (O'Donovan et al., 2015). Indeed, the 2019 report from the Global System for Mobile Communications suggested that there will be over 600 million unique subscribers to mobile networks by 2025 across sub-Saharan Africa, representing just over half of its total population (GSMA, 2020).

Importantly, in relation to CHW training and supervision, mHealth has been suggested to have a role in addressing two key challenges: first, the importance of just-in-time information for CHWs, including training, factual information, and decision support (including approaches supported by Artificial Intelligence); and second, addressing logistical challenges and barriers of geography and economic circumstance.

Yet, despite the technical and logistical benefits attached to mHealth facilitated training and supervision, less attention has been given to the pedagogical benefits of mHealth as a means of facilitating and supporting the delivery of training and supervision. Indeed, a 2018 systematic scoping review published by Winters and team reported that few mobile learning initiatives for CHWs are underpinned by educational research and theory (Winters et al., 2018b). The authors argue that the majority of mHealth training initiatives for CHWs adhere to over-simplified models of learning that fail to account for the complexities that emerge when new technologies are introduced into pedagogical practice. This led the authors to suggest that mHealth 'suffers from a reductionist view of learning that underestimates the complexities of the relationship between pedagogy and technology' (Winters et al., 2018b, p. 1). Instead they call for a greater level of interdisciplinary collaboration between the health- and education communities to incorporate a more critical educational perspective into the design and deployment of mobile learning projects for CHWs.

Similarly, the way in which technology mediated training and supervision for CHWs is evaluated has the potential to be radically reconceptualized. Prevailing approaches to studying educational technology have often focused on research questions related to 'what works?' This has generated positivist, instrumental studies to ascertain whether technologies have met prescribed educational objectives (Friesen, 2009). Experimental study designs have been favoured over other methodologies, while other forms of knowledge generated by practitioners remain ignored in favour of codified, standardized measures, reflecting entrenched policy concerns (Oliver & Conole, 2003). As CHW programmes continue to grow and evolve, and the demand for ongoing training and supervision comes into focus, we have an opportunity to address some of these often-overlooked concerns and reconceptualize CHW training and supervision.

CHW Voices and Structure of the Book

Ṣẹ̀yẹ Abímbọ́lá (2019, p. 4) poignantly observed that, 'the growing concerns about imbalances in authorship are a tangible proxy for concerns about power asymmetries in the production (and benefits) of knowledge in global health.' Much consideration has gone into the representation of authors and voices of CHWs in this book. While we, the editors of the book, are all from the same institution in a high-income country, our aim was to bring together global experts to share their experiences, balancing gender and LMIC representation as much as possible. To ensure that the voices of CHWs are fully represented, not just through their organizations, but also individually, a website accompanying this book will feature videos and interviews of CHWs about their experiences, roles, and challenges faced in their daily practice.

The book is divided into four key sections: CHW Training and Supervision, Education and Technology, Methodological Choice, and Ethics. In addition, we sought to enrich the book with real-life, practical case studies based on the work of organizations or research groups involved with CHWs.

Section One of the book focuses on *training and supervision,* and builds on the relationship between theory and practice, considering the increasing role of technology within this.

In Chapter 2, Raj Panjabi and his team outline the promise of digital health for supporting the training of CHWs, and importantly draw attention to the specific ways in which technology can help address learning needs. Framing their work from a WHO perspective, they note the need for a CHW curriculum, with technology-based learning at its core.

In Chapter 3, Dan Palazuelos and Sanjay Gadi explore how CHWs can be positioned to work within teams of health providers, so that investments in health systems yield greater returns in healthcare delivery with excellent and equitable outcomes. They discuss why CHWs are well positioned to represent community challenges and wisdom and outline what CHWs can do to offer new arenas for improving health outcomes.

In Chapter 4, James O'Donovan introduces different approaches to training and supervision of CHWs and reviews their evolution over time.

In Chapter 5, Beatrice Wasunna and Isaac Holeman discuss the work of Medic, a non-profit digital health organization, with operations in Nepal and more than a dozen other countries around the world. They explain the rationale behind the Medic's Community Health Toolkit and examine Medic's approach and challenges to implementation at scale.

Section Two explores the intersection of *technology and education* in the context of CHW training.

In Chapter 6, Shobhana Nagraj examines the evidence base for the pedagogical approaches used to design technology-enhanced learning (TEL) for CHWs and develops a six-step approach to designing a TEL-based training or supervision programme for CHWs, highlighting the importance of contextualizing CHW learning within the wider health system.

In Chapter 7, Jade Vu Henry examines how mobile phones can help move training programmes out of the classroom and into community settings where CHWs live and work. The chapter discusses what happens to 'learning' when training becomes 'mobile'. More specifically, it asks, what does it mean to 'learn' when the training for CHWs 'moves'.

Section Three investigates how *methodological choice* can contribute to social justice in CHW programmes and facilitate CHW training in an equitable way.

In Chapter 8, David Musoke looks at participatory approaches to train CHWs, evaluating strengths and weaknesses of prevalent participatory methods.

In Chapter 9, Promise Nduku, Nkululeko Tshabalala, Shona Putuka, Zafeer Ravat, and Laurenz Langer outline how taking a more systematic approach to developing a responsive evidence base that can inform research, policy, and practice on CHW training in LMICs can ultimately support the provision of more effective and equitable CHW programmes.

In Chapter 10, Celia Brown discusses the importance of evaluation in maximizing the impact of CHW training programmes. Whilst the author recognizes a number of different approaches to evaluation, the chapter sets out specific guidance on how to conduct systematic evaluations with a quantitative measure of effectiveness.

In Section Four, *ethical issues* arising from CHW training are discussed.

In Chapter 11, Maureen Kelley and Nigel Fancourt observe the way in which ethical culture is shaped and reinforced through education and supervision. The authors call for greater attention to the inherent worth of CHWs and draw attention to the importance of equipping CHWs to manage moral distress in their work through robust ethics planning and supervision.

In Chapter 12, the book's editors reflect on the challenges and opportunities identified in this volume, and highlight the ways forward proposed by the authors of this volume to shape new CHW-driven pedagogies.

References

Abímbólá, S. (2019). The foreign gaze: Authorship in academic global health. *BMJ Global Health*, 4, e002068.

Altobelli, L.C. (2017). Sharing histories—a transformative learning/teaching method to empower community health workers to support health behavior change of mothers. *Human Resources & Health*, 15(54). Available from: https://doi.org/10.1186/s12960-017-0231-2

Bahn, D. (2001). Social learning theory: Its application in the context of nurse education. *Nurse Education Today*, 21(2), 110–117.

Ballard, M., Madore, A., Johnson A., Keita, Y., Haag, E., Palazuelos, D., et al. (2018). *Concept Note: Community Health Workers*. Cambridge MA, Harvard Business Publishing.

Brackertz, N. (2007). ISR Working Paper Who is hard to reach and why? Available from: http://library.bsl.org.au/jspui/bitstream/1/875/1/Whois_htr.pdf

Ertmer, P.A. & Newby, T.J. (2013). Behaviorism, cognitivism, constructivism: Comparing critical features from an instructional design perspective. *Performance Improvement Quarterly*, 26(2), 43–71.

Freire, P. (1970). *Pedagogy of the Oppressed*. London, Continuum.

Friesen, N. (2009). *Re-thinking e-learning Research: Foundations, Methods, and Practices*. New York, Peter Lang.

Global Health Workforce Alliance (2010). *Global Experience of Community Health Workers for Delivery of Health Related Millennium Development Goals: A Systematic Review, Country Case Studies, and Recommendations for Integration into National Health Systems*. Geneva, World Health Organization.

Global Health Workforce Alliance (2013). Global health workforce crisis—key messages. Available from: https://www.who.int/workforcealliance/media/KeyMessages_3GF.pdf?ua=1 Global System for Mobile Communications (2020). The mobile economy—sub-Saharan African 2019. https://www.gsma.com/mobileeconomy/wp-content/uploads/2020/03/GSMA_MobileEconomy2020_SSA_Eng.pdf

Labrique, A.B., Vasudevan, L., Kochi, E., Fabricant, R., & Mehl, G. (2013). mHealth innovations as health system strengthening tools: 12 common applications and a visual framework. *Global health: Science and Practice*, 1(2), 160–171.

Lehmann, U. & Sanders, D. (2007). *Community Health Workers: What do We Know About Them? The State of the Evidence on Programmes, Activities, Costs and Impact on Health Outcomes of Using Community Health Workers*. Geneva, World Health Organization.

Ludwick, T., Turyakira, E., Kyomuhangi, T., Manalili, K., Robinson, S., & Brenner, J.L. (2018). Supportive supervision and constructive relationships with healthcare workers support CHW performance: Use of a qualitative framework to evaluate CHW programming in Uganda. *Human Resources for Health*, 16(1), 11. Available from: https://doi.org/10.1186/s12960-018-0272-1

Oliver, M., Geniets, A., Winters, N., Rega, I., & Mbae, S.M. (2015). What do community health workers have to say about their work, and how can this inform improved programme design? A case study with CHWs within Kenya. *Global Health Action*, 8(1)., doi: 10.3402/gha.v8.27168

Mathers, N. & Huang, Y.C. (2014). The future of general practice in China: from 'barefoot doctors' to GPs? *British Journal of General Practice*, 64(623), 270–271.

O'Donovan, J., Bersin, A., & O'Donovan, C. (2015). The effectiveness of mobile health (mHealth) technologies to train healthcare professionals in developing countries: A review of the literature. *BMJ Innovations*, 1(1), 33–36.

O'Donovan, J., Hamala, R., Namanda, A.S., Musoke, D., Ssemugabo, C., & Winters, N. (2020). 'We are the people whose opinions don't matter'. A photovoice study exploring challenges faced by community health workers in Uganda. *Global Public Health*, 15(3), 384–401.

Oliver, M. & Conole, G. (2003). Evidence-based practice and e-learning in Higher Education: Can we and should we? *Research Papers in Education*, 18(4), 385–397.

Perry, H. (2013). A brief history of community healthworker programs. https://www.mchip.net/sites/default/files/mchipfiles/02_CHW_History.pdf

Perry, H.B., Zulliger R., & Rogers, M.M. (2014). Community health workers in low-, middle-, and high-income countries: An overview of their history, recent evolution, and current effectiveness. *Annual Review of Public Health*, 35, 399–421.

Prinja, S., Jeet, G., Verma, R., Kumar, D., Bahuguna, P., Kaur, M., et al. (2014). Economic analysis of delivering primary health care services through community health workers in 3 North Indian states. *PLoS One*, 9, e91781. Available from: https://doi.org/10.1371/journal.pone.0091781.

Redick, C., Faich Dini, H.S., & Long, L.-A. (2014). *The Current State of CHW Training Programs in sub-Saharan Africa and South Asia: What We Know, What We Don't Know, and What We Need to do*. Virginia, One Million Community Health Workers Campaign, mPowering Frontline Health Workers.

Rifkin, S. (2017). *Community Health Workers*. In: S. Quah & W. Cockerham (Eds). *International Encyclopedia of Public Health* (Second Edition). Vol. 1. Amsterdam, Elsevier.

Rosenthal, M. & Greiner, J. (1982). The barefoot doctors of China: from political creation to professionalization. *Human Organization*, 41(4), 330–341.

Ruiz, Y., Matos, S., Kapadia, S., Islam, N., Cusack, A., Kwong, S., et al. (2012). Lessons learned from a community-academic initiative: The development of a core competency-based training for community-academic initiative community health workers. *American Journal of Public Health*, 102(12), 2372–2379.

Scott, K., Beckham, S.W., Gross, M., Pariyo, G., Rao, K.D., Cometto, G., et al. (2018). What do we know about community-based health worker programs? A systematic review of existing reviews on community health workers. *Human Resources for Health*, 16(1), 39. Available from: https://doi.org/10.1186/s12960-018-0304-x

Sfard, A. (1998). On two metaphors for learning and the dangers of choosing just one. *Educational Researcher*, 27(2), 4–13.

Sidel, V. (1968). Feldshers and feldsherism—the role and training of the feldsher in the USSR. *New England Journal of Medicine*, 278, 987–992.

Winters, N., Oliver, M., & Langer, L. (2017). Can mobile health training meet the challenge of 'measuring better'? *Comparative Education*, 53(1), 115–131.

Winters, N., Langer, L., & Geniets, A. (2018a). Scoping review assessing the evidence used to support the adoption of mobile health (mHealth) technologies for the education and training of community health workers (CHWs) in low-income and middle-income countries. *BMJ Open*, 8(7), e019827. Available from: doi:10.1136/bmjopen-2017-019827.

Winters, N., O'Donovan, J., & Geniets, A. (2018b). A new era for community health in countries of low and middle income? *Lancet Global Health*, 6(5), e489–e490.

World Health Organization (1978). International Conference on Primary Health Care. Declaration of Alma-Ata. In: Alma-Ata, USSR: World Health Organization. Available from: http://www.who.int/publications/almaata_declaration_en.pdf?ua=1

World Health Organization (2006). *Working Together for Health: The World Health Report 2006*. Geneva, World Health Organization.

World Health Organization (2007). *Community Health Workers: What do we Know About Them? The State of the Evidence on Programmes, Activities, Costs and Impact on Health Outcomes of Using Community Health Workers*. Geneva, World Health Organization.

World Health Organization (2018). *WHO Guideline on Health Policy and System Support to Optimize Community Health Worker Programmes*. Geneva, World Health Organization.

2

The Role of Technology in Supporting the Education of Community Health Workers and their Leaders

Raj Panjabi, Lesley-Anne Long, Michael Bailey, and Magnus Conteh

Introduction: The Community Health Worker

Over half the world lacks access to essential health services (WHO, 2019a). Many will never see a health worker in their entire lives. In rural communities, most of those who do will head directly to front-line health workers, often a community health worker (CHW). CHWs often represent the first point of contact for many individuals in low-income countries accessing health services. The WHO *Guideline on Health Policy and System Support to Optimize Community Health Worker Programs* (WHO, 2018, referred to as 'the CHW Guideline'), stated that: 'Governments, development partners, civil society organizations, and research and academic institutions have expressed a clear demand for scaling up CHW programs, and are committed to integrating CHW programs into health systems and harmonizing their actions accordingly' (p. 19).

This chapter briefly outlines the growing importance of (and focus on) the role of CHW programmes in low and middle-income countries (LMICs) and examines the underpinning principles for delivering effective pre-service clinical education and in-service training (to impart specific competencies) to CHWs. It considers the challenges and limits of current approaches, before going on to appraise the potential of technology to addresses these challenges. The chapter ends with recommendations for a global, co-ordinated approach to supporting the education of CHWs that uses the inherent scalability of digital technologies and has the promise to improve health outcomes for all.

Gaps in Community Health Worker Quality and Why Change Is Needed

The introduction of CHWs to provide accessible primary care, expanding in the last decades from preventive and promotive services, such as distributing contraceptives,

Raj Panjabi, Lesley-Anne Long, Michael Bailey, and Magnus Conteh, *The Role of Technology in Supporting the Education of Community Health Workers and their Leaders* In: *Training for Community Health.* Edited by: Anne Geniets, James O'Donovan, Laura Hakimi, and Niall Winters, Oxford University Press. © Oxford University Press 2021.
DOI: 10.1093/oso/9780198866244.003.0002

to include curative services such as integrated community case management of malaria, pneumonia, diarrhoea, malnutrition, and newborn sepsis management, has increased uptake of care in many areas of the world. The CHW Guideline acknowledges the range of healthcare services that CHWs provide to underserved populations and the role that CHWs play in situations of emergency, such as Ebola and other health shocks, as well as their contribution to reducing inequities in access to care (WHO, 2018, p.13).

CHWs' role in increasing access to health services has also, in some cases, improved quality of care. In some studies, caregivers of children receiving care from CHWs were more satisfied than with similar care delivered in a facility, particularly in relation to access, trust, and communication (Shaw et al., 2016). Like all healthcare providers, however, CHWs often face challenges in providing the quality of care that is needed to achieve the targeted individual and community health goals. In an observational study of trained and supervised CHWs in Tanzania, Baynes and colleagues found that while some areas of delivery were consistently high quality—such as assessment—in other cases, symptoms were missed and treatment was incorrect (26% of pneumonia and 29% of diarrhoea cases) (Baynes et al., 2018). The authors note that these quality gaps were often related to shortcomings in the supervision and stockouts of supplies.

There is a quality crisis in the delivery of community-oriented primary healthcare. Poor quality of care is associated with more deaths than access, with an estimated five million deaths due to poor quality among people using care and 3.6 million from lack of access (Kruk et al., 2018). Underlying causes of this quality gap can include lack of knowledge or skills, low levels of supervision or feedback, or inadequate supplies and equipment (Bagonza et al., 2014). In addition, local contextual factors including sociocultural norms, safety and security, and health system functioning (as well as the education) can influence CHW performance (Kok et al., 2015). Therefore, to improve the quality of care delivery, multifaceted approaches are needed. These include going beyond traditional training alone (Rowe et al., 2018), to ensure that the needed skills are not only developed but maintained through supportive supervision and education, along with system management to ensure that the supplies are provided on time and that the CHWs are salaried to provide the motivation and professionalism needed (WHO, 2018).

In January 2019, the World Health Organization (WHO) Executive Board took the important step in formally supporting and recognizing the value of CHWs as part of a diverse and sustainable health workforce skills mix. The Executive Board adopted a resolution introduced by the Governments of Ethiopia and Ecuador, entitled: 'Community health workers delivering primary healthcare: Opportunities and challenges'. The document, which builds on both countries' experience and the Declaration of Astana (WHO & UNICEF, 2018), underscores the importance of

CHWs as a vital health system component in providing primary healthcare services (WHO, 2019b).

State of the Knowledge of Pedagogy and Education Principles Relevant to CHWs and Supporting Programmes

Given the exceptional importance of CHWs, a critical question remains: why are so many still profoundly undertrained? The consequences of this severe under-training of CHWs contributes to the deaths of millions of children under five every year, as well as to the hundreds of thousands of women who continue to die as a result of pregnancy or childbirth (UNICEF, 2018; WHO, 2019a). All too often, undertrained CHWs do not know how to intervene appropriately. Training CHWs in a way that is appropriate (relevant to their context and level of education) and cost effective therefore promises to deliver significantly improved health outcomes for populations in LMICs and a better quality of life for individuals, families, and communities.

Other chapters in this volume discuss pedagogies appropriate for use in CHW training. Aligned to this, in a systematic review of learning methodologies for health worker training, Bluestone et al. (2013):

> Identified that didactic instruction, such as relying on reading and lecture, often results in no to low learning outcome. In contrast, the use of interactive, practice-heavy techniques, such as clinical simulation, case-based learning, hands-on practice with anatomic models, and immediate feedback on performance, results in better learning outcomes. In addition, repeated frequency is preferable to one-time training interventions; workplace learning may be superior for skill acquisition, and multiple media modes of delivery can be used to deliver training more efficiently.
>
> (Jhpiego, 2016, p. 1)

Moreover, a teacher-centric approach is hard to scale. Given the critical shortage of CHWs and the failure of traditional education and training models (e.g. see Getachew et al., 2019), LMICs are therefore being driven to invest in approaches that combine classroom instruction with distance learning, including using mobile devices to make training content more widely available and in an accessible multi-media format designed for the CHW that can supplement and enhance existing education and training of CHWs.

As detailed in Chapter 1, during the last decade, digital technologies have demonstrated their potential as capacity building mechanisms to support health workforce development in LMICs, including for training, supervising, and paying CHWs.

The Promise of Digital Health

What does this technological advancement mean for community health pro-grammes and CHW education and training? Connectivity in remote and rural areas remains challenging and this is unlikely to change soon. Yet despite this, many coun-tries see digital health as an important resource for their health workers, including CHWs. The potential of technologies is also recognized at a global level. In 2018, governments unanimously adopted a World Health Assembly resolution calling on WHO to develop a global strategy on digital health to support national efforts to achieve universal health coverage (WHO, 2019c). Later in the same year, WHO published a comprehensive classification of digital health interventions (Shrivastava & Shrivastava, 2019), highlighting ways in which digital technology offers oppor-tunities for health workers to undergo training, collect data more efficiently, make evidence-informed decisions, and support other functions to improve healthcare service and delivery. And in April 2019, WHO released new recommendations on ways that countries can use digital technology to improve people's health and essen-tial services (WHO, 2019d), including recommendations that are relevant to CHW education and training as well as community health programming. These recom-mendations regarding the use of digital technology and mobile devices for health services include: birth and death notifications, stock notification and commodity management, client-to-provider and provider-to-provider telemedicine, health worker decision support, and provision of training and educational content to health workers.

Digital technologies clearly have the potential to help address problems such as ac-cess to services, health worker training and decision-making. However, the promise of digital health has led to: 'proliferation of short-lived implementations and an over-whelming diversity of digital tools, with a limited understanding of their impact on health systems and people's well-being' (WHO, 2019e). This fragmentation and short-termism is exacerbated by a lack of investment in building digital health capacity within the health system more broadly; this leaves countries without the expertise they need to design, implement, and support digital health systems at scale (and sus-tainably) to improve health outcomes.

The potential role of technology in CHW programming and CHW education and training is therefore currently poised delicately between the rhetoric of what's pos-sible and the reality on the ground. 'Digital health has the potential to help address problems such as distance and access, but still shares many of the underlying chal-lenges faced by health system interventions... including insufficient training, infra-structural limitations, etc... These considerations need to be addressed in addition to the specific implementation requirements introduced by digital health' (WHO, 2019e, p. 77cc.).

How Technology Can Address the Challenges and Help Meet Learning Needs

Decades of research have affirmed that, as long as certain conditions are met, distance learning can perform as well as face-to-face learning (Zhao et al., 2005; Means et al., 2010). One of those conditions includes access to face-to-face learning, suggesting that a blended learning approach is perhaps a better characterization of an effective use of technology for improving the learning experience (McCutcheon et al., 2014). A more recent systematic review and meta-analysis focusing on the use of mobile technology for training health professionals concluded that 'm-learning is as effective as traditional learning or possibly more so' (Dunleavy et al., 2019, p. 1). The use of mobile devices for learning is also ideally suited for the low-dose, high-frequency approach to training delivery advocated by Bluestone et al. (2013), in particular when complemented with face-to-face learning to the point where it can be regarded as a truly blended learning approach. At the same time, a new Cochrane systematic review concluded: 'general claims of [mobile learning for health professionals] as inherently more effective than traditional learning may be misleading' (Vaona et al., 2018). This recent systematic review of e-learning for health professionals, started with 3464 identified studies which resulted in only 16 studies that met the inclusion criteria. None of the 16 studies were conducted in an African country (Vaona et al., 2018). If there is uncertainty around conclusions about e-learning effectiveness for healthcare in modern settings with a robust telecommunications infrastructure, more context specific research may be necessary in settings of unreliable connectivity involving health workers in rural communities.

What is fairly certain, is that the effective use of the technology is context dependent and one should consider other factors, such as cost savings, the inaccessibility of training in remote areas, reduction in the need of printed material, etc., when evaluating the proposed use of mobile or distance education (Vaona et al., 2018). The Guideline contains recommendations around pre-service training related to competencies, recruitment, and modalities for delivery to enhance the effectiveness of CHWs on health outcomes. Despite the added value these recommendations would provide if adopted, they fail to acknowledge the working reality of many CHWs, where unplanned experiential learning is often the norm, driven by necessity. For example, there will be instances where a CHW will be unprepared to deal with an issue in his/her day-to-day work and require access to reliable 'just-in-time' information. This may be related to data collection, a community education day, or other CHW activities. Digital health has a significant role to play in being able to support that CHW by providing an immediate link to content relevant to the activity s/he is undertaking. This means preparing for the eventual integration of training content with related data collection, diagnostic applications, telehealth for referrals, and opportunities for peer-based learning. For it is not sufficient for a CHW to know the background on Family Planning (FP) commodities, for example, to provide actionable advice for their clients. They also need to know a client's medical history (available through a digital client registry), the availability of a particular FP commodity (available through a digital logistics management information system), and, ideally, the effectiveness of that commodity within a given context (available through an Artificial Intelligence (AI)-based decision support tool). It is this integration of related technology (and the use of AI in decision-making) (Liu et al., 2019) which can, if properly executed, help compensate for gaps in training.

Unfortunately, this interdependence among digital tools designed for information dissemination (such as m-learning), data collection, and decision support has yet to be fully acknowledged. Conceptually, the recognition of interdependence and the need for interoperability between heterogeneous health systems has been long-standing (Cardoso et al., 2018). However, this need has not been sufficiently acted upon in operations, particularly in community health settings, despite the growing use of open Application Programming Interfaces (APIs) and data standards (such as Health Level Seven [HL7]).

Consider the interdependence between the content available from a worker's educational resource, the information the workers then provide to address the needs of specific clients, and whether they have the competency to dispense and act on the right information. Planning for integration with client and workforce registries becomes critical when bearing in mind how to ease the burden for health workers who have the responsibility of tracking their own clients, ensuring their profiles and work history are up to date, and accessing relevant content for their own education as well as the community population they serve. However, the implications of not coordinating the creation and implementation of digital educational content with the integration of other digital health tools is most profound in the case of decision support, which is increasingly provided through AI. The two airline crashes involving the 737 MAX 800 aircraft provide a stark reminder of the implications of failing to ensure the training provided to humans gives them an adequate understanding of the basis for decisions provided by automated support systems (Fallows, 2019). Whether that support is provided in the course of flying an aircraft or in support of diagnosing the health conditions of patients.

Ideally the treatment protocols and training materials used by the health workforce should serve as the basis for any algorithms used for the development of AI solutions used in health worker decision-making. In this way when there are changes in guidelines/protocols there is a system in place that can implement those changes for both the human training materials/curriculum as well as the algorithms serving as the basis for AI solutions.

This is not just a question of technical consistency between two sources of health services (a trained health worker and the logic of an AI application based on training data); it is also a question of trust. If a health worker doesn't understand the basis of a decision provided from an external tool—and especially if that tool's decision is inconsistent with the training s/he received—s/he is less likely to trust the tool for future support. In reality, some AI-based decision support tools can derive a diagnosis or recommendation from highly optimized algorithms that depend on contextualized training data. Although published and 'transparent', this evidence can be impenetrable to the health worker. Emerging data protection standards such as European Union's (EU) General Data Protection Regulation (GDPR) provide openings to bridge this gap by providing legal rights for users to request explanations for why certain decisions are made. Combining this principle with a new movement known as Explainable AI (which refers to methods and techniques in the application of artificial intelligence technology such that the results of the solution can be understood by human experts) (Wikipedia, 2019) can help prevent mistrust or provide a means for tracing a source of bias in the logic of an application.

One way of reducing a dependence on experts to explain the decision-making process of external applications after these programmes are implemented is to engage with domain experts from the beginning. By working directly with medical personnel from the start (and not just through interviews), with the intent of ensuring consistency between materials used for training in human and machine learning, problems around trust can be addressed from the start. The advantages of this approach are stressed in an article by Keitel and D'Acremont (2018, p. 853): 'This process [of validating the algorithms] could be greatly facilitated through the development of an interface which automates the transformation of the traditional visual decision tree into programming source code, thereby minimizing errors and allowing more clinicians to participate in and review the algorithm design.' Even without this logical alignment between the resources that provide the basis for the content used in AI decision support and the source material used for training the average health worker, certain categories of decision support tools collectively known as electronic clinical decision algorithms (eCDA) have already 'shown early promise in improving the management of febrile children in primary care while increase[ing] the rational use of diagnostics and antimicrobials' (Keitel & D'Acremont, 2018). AI can also provide support in overcoming the complexity associated with evaluating symptoms, test results, disease classifications, and other factors simultaneously to detect patients with serious bacterial infections and thus avoid the irrational overprescribing of antibiotics (Keitel, 2019).

For private and public institutions responsible for training a health workforce, the transition to a completely digital representation (i.e. elimination of hard copy job aids and manuals) and the generation of evidence to support this transition will take time. What has become increasingly evident is the need to coordinate the development (or adaptation) of job -aids, multimedia production, data collection tools, and algorithm development (for both hard copy and AI based decision support) in conjunction with a primary healthcare (PHC) curriculum in order to ensure that all these components actually complement one another. Without this coordination one runs the risk of simply layering the tools and multimedia content on top of a curriculum designed without any of these additional components in mind. Unless the curriculum is properly revised to reflect the use of multimedia and additional digital tools the result is a fragmented tool set and an unstable foundation for blended learning.

Bringing It All Together

It is time to capitalize on two important global trends: the recognition of education and health in terms of a Sustainable Development Goal (SDG), and acknowledgement of the importance of CHWs as a primary means to achieve Universal Health Coverage (UHC). Coupled with the efficiencies of digital technology and growing consensus around the commonality of the PHC curriculum, there is a compelling rationale for a globally representative and locally adaptable CHW curriculum which can be contextualized for local need as required. This global content would fulfil the traditional definition of a 'global public good' (GPG). The GPG model promises potential benefits to all countries; content would be available for governments to draw from and (working with non-governmental organizations (NGOs) and other partners) localize to address health priorities at a national or even regional level. The GPG model may also be the only way to bring about a sustainable, globally scalable solution that can address the need for a trained and skilled community health workforce across LMICs.

There are two elements at the centre of this GPG model. First, is the establishment of a globally representative, locally adaptable PHC curriculum. The second is the integration of that content with a process for updating treatment protocols and guidelines (Fairall et al., 2018). With embedded multimedia content (which has been designed for rapid contextual adaptation), this curriculum can be delivered in digital form to CHWs via their mobile devices. This approach allows each country to assume ownership by providing access to a networked library of educational resources, a learning management platform, and a process to customize the content according to their local context and disease burden.

Many LMICs cannot support such a process on their own and global institutions are recognizing the need to play a more substantive role in strengthening each country's health systems. In a speech presented at the first Prix Galien International in Africa in 2018, WHO Director-General Dr Tedros Ghebreyesus admitted that: 'health systems and health security are two sides of the same coin. We are only as strong as our weakest link' (Ghebreyesus, 2018). Dr Tedros has proposed a more activist role for WHO, referring directly to the new partnership between WHO and the Institute for Health Metrics and Evaluation (IHME), the Global Burden of Disease's scientific centre. Dr Tedros believes that the Global Burden of Disease centre can strengthen WHO by providing some of the most reliable data for the agency to use in its proposed country consultations.

There is a potentially rich, interdependent relationship between a country's digitally empowered community health workforce and the predictive capacity of IHME which relies on reliable data sources to create robust models of each country's disease burden. By equipping a country's community health workforce with basic functionality—for example around death notification and digital tracking of patients'/ clients' health status using mobile devices—a previously unavailable source of reliable, timely, aggregated, and anonymized information related to mortality and morbidity of a country's population becomes available to IHME for analysis and timely feedback for each country. This will help countries define training and resource priorities by disease burden. With only slight modifications in data collection and storage, this information can also inform a best practices database through the collection of data related to health worker performance and related training content to assess what worked and what did not in improving health worker use and knowledge of content and ultimately improvement in client health.

Through the creation of a dynamic process that leverages the common elements of the PHC curriculum, embeds adaptable multimedia, and is periodically recalibrated to reflect a country's real individual disease burden, a sustainable, digitally based content delivery system for health training is achievable. By approaching the challenge of health delivery in the last mile as a global one—where global institutions, are actively engaged in the process of content delivery and health worker training—the gap between the validation of new treatments and guidelines and the adaptation to practice on the front line can be reduced from years to weeks.

The Academy Initiative

A sober appraisal of the state of health service provision at the front lines in most LMICs exposes:

- An unaffordable CHW curriculum and training development process that fails to keep pace with changes in global or local clinical evidence and protocols and disease burden.
- Delays in releasing and communicating evidence-based practical knowledge equitably to all CHWs; contributing to a performance and quality gap in service delivery and delaying action on events involving potential epidemics.
- A general failure to leverage the interoperability of delivery technologies and effectiveness of multimedia content, due to a fragmented and duplicative digital ecosystem.

In 2017 Last Mile Health (LMH) launched a new initiative, the Community Health Academy ('the Academy') to address these and other critical issues relating to community health programmes and to modernize and re-imagine the education of CHWs and health systems leaders for the digital age. The focus of this initiative is on helping to build a skilled, digitally literate health workforce at the community level, as well as supporting the development of cadres of health leaders (e.g. policymakers, managers, and supervisors) who are involved in community health systems planning and implementation. Working with global, regional, and national partners, including governments, health practitioners, academics, private sector organizations, donors, foundations, and United Nation entities, this initiative will leverage the potential of digital technology to contribute to the training of thousands of CHWs and the leaders who support them. Working in a variety of countries, the mission of LMH is to transform the lives and health outcomes of millions of people by 2030.

To achieve these goals, LMH is working with ministries to develop Clinical Education (CE) programmes for CHWs. These CE programmes will provide multimedia educational content that can be used to provide a blended learning approach towards CHW training. The approach is intended to reinforce—not replace—existing training (in-person and digital) programmes. These programmes will support refresher and enhanced training for CHWs to improve their competencies when delivering health services and their understanding of when and how to refer patients to higher level facilities. More than 3500 CHWs and nurse/midwife supervisors are currently equipped with malaria and malnutrition digital content in Liberia in an ongoing deployment, while agreements have been reached with ministry officials in Ethiopia, Sierra Leone, and Uganda to also initiate deployment in those countries.

Working with Ministries of Health and other partners, LMH—together with affiliates in West and Central Africa, East and Southern Africa—will anticipate priority CHW training needs in sub-Saharan Africa. Existing content will be re-used or adapted and, where there are gaps, new content will be commissioned to address those training needs. The content will be delivered to CHWs via mobile devices through a platform which also provides assessment activities. This model will enable training programmes to reach CHWs even in rural or remote areas and will mitigate the need for CHWs to leave their communities to attend trainings for long periods of time. The model will also enable the supervisors/trainers of CHWs to remotely monitor their progress via dashboards which capture CHW frequency and length of use of the content, as well as their quizzes and test scores. Using this information, governments can be supported to develop assessed learning pathways and to use CHW competency scores to accredit CHWs.

LMH's Health Systems Leadership Development (HSLD) Programme was launched Organized as a global classroom for health systems leaders by health systems leaders the programme focuses on community health leaders and programme implementers. Launched in 2019, the HSLD Programme will provide an open source suite of high-quality online courses supported by communities of practice (CoPs). CoPs are being established (both on- and offline) for HSLD alumni, as well as for policymakers, managers, and supervisors, to promote peer-to-peer learning and support the application of learning to the field.

The first leadership course: *Strengthening Community Health Worker Programs to Deliver Primary Health Care*, went 'live' in May 2019, with over 11,000 learners from over 180 countries enrolling in the course. The course features case studies taught by public sector health systems leaders who have built exemplar programmes in Bangladesh, Ethiopia, and Liberia, alongside lectures from global experts from WHO,

USAID, the Global Fund for AIDS, TB, and Malaria, and the Global Financing Facility at the World Bank Group.

The HSLD curriculum is aligned with WHO's building blocks of effective health systems—leadership and governance, health workforce, service delivery, health information, supply chain and operations, and health financing—adding in community engagement as a critical component. The suite of courses, created in partnership with a faculty network of leading community health innovators from around the world, will explore linkages between these building blocks and include case studies from in-country experts. LMH's goal is to train at least 15,000 health leaders by 2021.

Conclusion

'Digital technologies provide concrete opportunities to tackle health systems challenges, and thereby offer the potential to enhance the coverage and quality of health practices and services'

WHO Digital Health Guideline (WHO, 2019e, p. iii).

It is now widely acknowledged that digital technologies have a role to play in advancing UHC and improving the quality of care delivered, even care at the last mile, delivered by CHWs. WHO specifically recommends the provision of learning and training content via mobile devices, while cautioning that traditional methods of delivering health education and post-certificate training should not be replaced.

This chapter suggests that given the increasing recognition that health is a global phenomenon, combined with the inherent scalability of digital technologies, there is a unique opportunity to solve problems on a global scale. Starting with the CHW curriculum being adopted as a global public resource, the proposed approach challenges the present governance and procurement model which 'carves up the map' according to an outdated set of donor priorities. The vast majority of content for training CHWs is held in common around the world (a greater percentage held in common on a regional basis) and is easily adaptable to context, culture, and language. The success of WHO's integrated management of childhood illness (IMCI) content is one illustration of the use of global content for health workers (Horwood et al., 2019). The technology used to disseminate the content can be scaled globally. It also enables a more engaging and user-centric approach to learning through the use of multi-media content, quizzes, and other interactive materials, as well as supporting 'just-in-time' learning for CHWs in the field, wanting a reminder about a clinical or behaviour change intervention. The technology also provides a means to rapidly update treatment protocols and adapt them for context (once the processes to do this are in place). Finally, the training received, and the data collected by CHWs around disease prevalence, can be relayed back into a global cycle of evaluation and then translated into practice at a rate many times faster than the present. Too often, a GPG remains an abstract notion;

what we're proposing is that if the underlying collective action problem is solved, a robust process for preparing the front lines of a country's health workforce exists.

The governance and procurement model that presently drives the development of national training curricula is the same governance and procurement model that leads to a fragmented approach towards the deployment of software solutions for the healthcare worker. These solutions are built around common software functions—data collection and information dissemination—that can be characterized as commodities. Yet like curricula, they are adopted by countries in an uncoordinated manner and often without regard for their interdependence and commonality. It is the CHWs' access to the information they need which should define these tools and relationships. If the CHW needs to know the fundamentals around nutrition, for example, s/he should be equipped with content that gives him/her the knowledge to recognize whether a child is malnourished and content that effectively communicates to a client the steps to remedy the situation. The specific functionality of the related data collection and decision support tools that can assist in the determination of a mother and child's nutritional health should also be based on those specific information requirements. Providing these digital tools as separate, unintegrated, applications—where the basis for the design differs from one tool to the next and is not aligned with the content and training provided to the health worker—simply makes a CHW's job and sustainability of this digitized health system more difficult. Therefore, like a national training curriculum, there needs to be an integrated digital tool set—defined by the health worker's information requirements, which would also qualify as a global public good.

There is a growing urgency to move beyond small-scale, pilot style demonstration CHW projects towards widespread, sustainable community health workforce systems. With the increasing ubiquity of smartphones and tablets and the expansion of functionalities available on these devices, together with a global commitment to integrate a common, adaptable curriculum, there is now the potential to achieve health workforce improvements, not only at the CHW programme level but across the whole health system.

References

Bagonza, J., Kibira, S., & Rutebemberwa, E. (2014). Performance of community health workers managing malaria, pneumonia and diarrhoea under the community case management programme in central Uganda: A cross sectional study. *Malaria Journal*, 13(1), 367.

Baynes, C., Mboya, D., Likasi, S., Maganga, D., Pemba, S., Baraka, J., et al. (2018). Quality of sick child-care delivered by community health workers in Tanzania. *International Journal of Health Policy and Management*, 7(12), 1097–1109.

Bluestone, J., Johnson, P., Fullerton, J., Carr, C., Alderman, J., & BonTempo, J. (2013). Effective in-service training design and delivery: Evidence from an integrative literature review. *Human Resources for Health*, 11(1), 51.

Cardoso, L., Marins, F., Quintas, C., Portela, F., Santos, M., Abelha, A., et al. (2018). Interoperability in healthcare. *Health Care Delivery and Clinical Science*, 689–714.

Dunleavy, G., Nikolaou, C., Nifakos, S., Atun, R., Law, G., & Tudor Car, L. (2019). Mobile digital education for health professions: Systematic review and meta-analysis by the Digital Health Education Collaboration. *Journal of Medical Internet Research*, 21(2), e12937.

Fairall, L., Cornick, R., & Bateman, E. (2018). Empowering frontline providers to deliver universal primary healthcare using the practical and approach to care kit. *BMJ Global Health*, 3, bmjgh-2018-k4451rep.

Fallows, J. (2019). Here's what was on the record about problems with the 737 Max. *The Atlantic*. Available from: https://www.theatlantic.com/notes/2019/03/heres-what-was-on-the-record-about-problems-with-the-737-max/584791/

Getachew, T., Mekonnen, S., Yitayal, M., Persson, L., & Berhanu, L. (2019). Health extension workers' diagnostic accuracy for common childhood illnesses in four regions of Ethiopia: A cross- sectional study. *Acta Paediatrica*, 108(11), 2100–2106.

Ghebreyesus, T. (2018). Opening speech at Prix Galien International. Available from: https://www.who.int/dg/speeches/2018/prix-galien-international/en/

Horwood, C., Voce, A., Vermaak, K., Rollins, N., & Qazi, S. (2009). Experiences of training and implementation of integrated management of childhood illness (IMCI) in South Africa: A qualitative evaluation of the IMCI case management training course. *BMC Pediatrics*, 9(1), 62.

Jhpiego, (2016). Low Dose, High Frequency: A learning approach to improve health workforce competence, confidence, and performance. *LDHF Briefer*. Available from: https://hms.jhpiego.org/wp-content/uploads/2016/08/LDHF_briefer.pdf

Keitel, K. (2019). Biomarkers to improve rational antibiotic use in low-resource settings. *Lancet Global Health*, 7(1), e14–e15.

Keitel, K. & D'Acremont, V. (2018). Electronic clinical decision algorithms for the integrated primary care management of febrile children in low-resource settings: Review of existing tools. *Clinical Microbiology and Infection*, 24(8), 845–855.

Kok, M.C., Kane, S.S., Tulloch, O., Ormel, H., Theobald, S., Dieleman, M., et al. (2015). How does context influence performance of community health workers in low- and middle-income countries? Evidence from the literature. *Health Resource Policy and Systems*, 13, 13.

Kruk, M., Gage, A., Arsenault, C., Jordan, K., Leslie, H., Roder-DeWan, S., et al. (2018). High-quality health systems in the Sustainable Development Goals era: Time for a revolution. *Lancet Global Health*, 6(11), e1196–e1252.

Liu, X., Faes, L., Kale, A., Wagner, S., Fu, D., Bruynseels, A., et al. (2019). A comparison of deep learning performance against health-care professionals in detecting diseases from medical imaging: A systematic review and meta-analysis. *Lancet Digital Health*, 1(6), e271–e297.

McCutcheon, K., Lohan, M., Traynor, M., & Martin, D. (2014). A systematic review evaluating the impact of online or blended learning vs. face-to-face learning of clinical skills in undergraduate nurse education. *Journal of Advanced Nursing*, 71(2), 255–270.

Means, B., Toyama, Y., Murphy, R., Bakia, M., & Jones, K. (2010). *Evaluation of Evidence-Based Practices in Online Learning: A Meta-Analysis and Review of Online Learning Studies Center for Technology in Learning*. Available from: www.ed.gov/about/offices/list/opepd/ppss/reports.html.

Rowe, A.K., Rowe, S.Y., Peters, D.H., Holloway, K.A., Chalker, J., & Ross-Degnan, D. (2018). Effectiveness of strategies to improve health-care provider practices in low-income and middle-income countries: A systematic review. *Lancet Global Health*, 6(11), 1163–e1175.

Shaw, B., Abdi, M., Asadhi, E., Owuor, K., Cohen, C., Onono, M., et al. (2016). Perceived quality of care of community health worker and facility-based health worker management of pneumonia in children under 5 years in Western Kenya: A cross-sectional multidimensional study. *American Journal of Tropical Medicine and Hygiene*, 94(5), 1170–1176.

Shrivastava, S. & Shrivastava, P. (2019). Digital interventions to strengthen the health sector: World Health Organization. *Digital Medicine*, 5(2), 90.

UNICEF (2019). *Levels and Trends in Child Mortality 2019*. Available from: https://www.unicef.org/reports/levels-and-trends-child-mortality-report-2019

Vaona, A., Banzi, R., Kwag, K., Rigon, G., Cereda, D., Pecoraro, V., et al. (2018). E-learning for health professionals. *Cochrane Database of Systematic Reviews 2018*, Issue 1. Art. No.: CD011736.

Wikipedia (2019). *Explainable Artificial Intelligence*. Available from: https://en.wikipedia.org/wiki/Explainable_artificial_intelligence

World Health Organization (2018). *WHO Guideline on Health Policy and System Support to Optimize Community Health Worker Programmes*. Geneva, World Health Organization.

World Health Organization (2019a). *Maternal Mortality*. Available from: https://www.who.int/news-room/fact-sheets/detail/maternal-mortality

World Health Organization (2019b). *Resolution on Community Health Workers to be considered at the upcoming World Health Assembly*. Available from: https://www.who.int/hrh/news/2019/community-health-workers-resolution-at-wha/en/

World Health Organization (2019c). *Health Workforce at the Seventy-second World Health Assembly*. Available from: https://www.who.int/hrh/news/2019/hw-72nd-wha/en/

World Health Organization (2019d). *WHO Releases First Guideline on Digital Health Interventions*. Available from: https://www.who.int/news-room/detail/17-04-2019-who-releases-first-guideline-on-digital-health-interventions

World Health Organization (2019e). *Recommendations on Digital Interventions for Health Systems Strengthening*. Available from: https://www.who.int/reproductivehealth/publications/digital-interventions-health-system-strengthening/en/

World Health Organization & UNICEF (2018). *Declaration of Astana*. Available from: https://www.who.int/docs/default-source/primary-health/declaration/gcphc-declaration.pdf

Zhao, Y., Lei, J., Yan, B., Lai, C., & Tan, H.S. (2005). What makes the difference? A practical analysis of research on the effectiveness of distance education. *Teachers College Record*, 107(8), 1836–1884.

3
Learning How Not to Train the Community Out of the Community Health Workers

Daniel Palazuelos and Sanjay Gadi

What CHWs Do

Community Health Workers (CHWs) are indispensable for the future of health-care delivery and the strengthening of healthcare systems. The capacities they are equipped to work in, however, will largely depend on how health system architects position CHWs, and how their training prepares them to do that job. A common strategy that started during the AIDS crisis but was further developed during the Millennium Development Goals era has been to shift medical tasks normally reserved for nurses and doctors to CHWs. The benefits of this approach are numerous, such as increased access to some life-saving interventions. But if CHWs are positioned simply as a 'low-cost solution' to the human resources crisis, then opportunities to leverage their unique skills, address disparities and inequities in care, and improve health outcomes will be lost. This chapter will explore how CHWs can best be trained and positioned to provide new functionality to a health system. Specifically, in this chapter, we will explore:

1) How CHWs can be positioned to *work within teams* of health providers so that investments in health systems yield greater returns in healthcare delivery with *excellent and equitable outcomes.*
2) Why CHWs should be positioned to *represent community challenges, and wisdom,* so that both the health system and community benefit.
3) What CHWs can do to offer *new arenas for improving health outcomes*, often surpassing previous benchmarks at a fraction of the cost.

This book is about training CHWs, and the premise of this chapter is that CHWs learn more about how to do their jobs through the quality of the health system in which they work and their position in it, than in classrooms alone. Any lessons taught explicitly will be easily washed away by implicit messages received during everyday

Daniel Palazuelos and Sanjay Gadi, *Learning How Not to Train the Community Out of the Community Health Workers* In: *Training for Community Health.* Edited by: Anne Geniets, James O'Donovan, Laura Hakimi, and Niall Winters, Oxford University Press. © Oxford University Press 2021. DOI: 10.1093/oso/9780198866244.003.0003

workflow—whether a patient is received with compassion or blame during a referral, whether a supervisor mentors with respect or paternalism, etc. All of this is the 'hidden curriculum' that we have experienced; it is better considered in an honest light and planned for directly.

CHWs Can Do So Much More

The current enthusiasm for CHWs is similar to that expressed in the post-Alma-Ata Conference period. Unlike that first round of national CHW programmes in the 1980s, however, this new round of CHW programming is being bolstered by funding sources previously not available, such as the Global Fund for AIDS, tuberculosis, and malaria, and ambitious healthcare movements, such as the push for universal health coverage. Through both of these periods, the appeal of the CHW has been about what they add to a traditional health system comprised of doctors, nurses, pharmacists, etc. For most, that appeal is based on the CHWs' position in the community and their knowledge of the local context; for others, the lower cost of their labour is the main appeal. Yet, underpinning the CHW movement has been a more complex issue: that of vulnerability and pathologic social stratification. Put simply, poverty makes you sick. A lack of access to healthy food, shelter, education, and jobs makes people ill, as does the sense of being separate and inferior, if not disparaged.

Many of the earliest practitioners of community health were driven primarily by the desire to address these inequities, such as the team that wrote the famous CHW training manual *Where There Is No Doctor*, and Paolo Freire, the Brazilian educator whose book *Pedagogy of the Oppressed* taught how education can be an instrument of oppression, or a revolutionary act (Werner et al., 1993; Freire, 2018). David Warner famously questioned if CHWs were to be 'liberators' of their communities, equipped to effectively confront the social determinants of disease that were making them sick, or 'lackeys' for health systems, subordinate to decisions made in a conversation that did not include them. History has given him a clear answer: CHWs are now largely positioned as 'lackeys,' since they are rarely given power to set priorities or control budgets, and many times are not even invited in any substantive way to the meetings and conferences held to determine their future work.

Even the local community health leadership of projects in impoverished countries aren't positioned equitably in the publications that demonstrate successes, when compared to their partners from the global north (Schneider & Maleka, 2018). The reasons behind this are multifactorial, including how rhetoric around revolutionary action was viewed during the cold war, how leftist movements in the geopolitically powerful northern countries, especially the USA, succumbed to a steady shift towards centrist/conservative policies, and how remnants of colonialism continue to exact their influence in how global health is practised daily. As such, CHWs are the pawns in the chess game of global health; they are on the front line (i.e. they take on great risk to themselves and their families), they have limited movement (i.e. they are not recognized internationally, so they cannot seek employment in other markets such as doctors and nurses can), and they are the most expendable (i.e. in many contexts, they are afforded no worker protections and can therefore be cut during even the smallest fluctuations in health budgets).

All this is not to say that CHWs are so disempowered that they are unable to con- tribute substantively to their communities—there are many examples where they pro- vide tremendous value to health systems at a fraction of the cost of other investments. Presently, the most common tasks undertaken by CHWs centre around health pro- motion, treatment support for diseases such as tuberculosis (TB), and maternal-child health interventions such as direct treatment of malaria, diarrhoea, and pneumonia in children under five years old (Scott et al., 2018). This latter medical protocol is known as the Integrated Community Case Management of childhood illness (iCCM). In small demonstration projects, iCCM has led to clinically important results, and most experts predict that this model will achieve similar efficacy in large popula- tions if brought to scale (however, this has yet to be definitively demonstrated as of 2020) (Scott et al., 2018; Sadruddin et al., 2019) The fact that iCCM has not always been successful at scale is more of an indictment of health system architects than of the CHWs' labour; if larger healthcare system strengthening efforts, such as supply chain management and quality care improvement in referral networks, are not funded along with the deployment of CHWs armed with rapid-diagnostic tests and treat- ment algorithms, then their efficacy can be systematically stunted. Experiences from smaller countries such as Rwanda, which deployed a massive CHW programme along with a concerted effort to fund and build a robust health system around those CHWs, have seen heartening drops in under-five mortality; from 2000 to 2011 in Rwanda, the probability that a child would die by the age of five years decreased by 70.4% (Farmer et al., 2013). This was below half of the regional average and approached the global mean. Although it is difficult to tease out the relative contributions of multiple dif- ferent factors, such as economic growth and the broader influence of a government that can effectively deploy health programmes, most agree that the CHW programme played an important role in these changes.

Other smaller sub-national experiences show that important alterations to the iCCM protocol can drive even greater impact and do so even faster. Such an example was shown in Mali by a non-governmental organization (NGO) named Muso (see case study in Appendix) using what they call the 'proactive-CCM' protocol. Mali is a large landlocked Francophone country in West Africa, that has a proud history of once being part of the powerful Mali Empire, but of late has been suffering from years of colonialism, desertification, and political turmoil. Muso is a 501c3 (US nonprofit) global health organization that was founded in 2005 by Malian and American collab- orators, and that partners closely with the government and local communities. The 'pro-CCM' protocol was developed by the team at Muso to reduce child mortality and improve early access to care. It incorporates a variety of inputs to achieve even greater results, most notably proactive case finding and treatment in the patients' houses (as opposed to passive case finding where clinicians wait in health centres for patients to arrive, despite the fact that referrals to health centres represent important barriers, with queues, travel costs, and opportunity costs), as well as referrals for free care at strengthened government clinics for severe cases that cannot be treated safely at home (Muso n.d.). One analysis showed that this approach reduced under-five mortality from one in every seven children under five years of age, to 1 in 142 (Johnson et al., 2018). This is a mortality rate of 7 deaths for every 1000 live births—a rate comparable to what can be expected in the Global North. However, this is not simply a workflow question that produces unprecedented results; instead, most proCCM investments occur in improving the staffing, equipment, infrastructure at primary care facilities, and in making sure that all medicines and services are provided with no user fees.

The relevance of such a proactive approach for other disorders, such as chronic diseases, has yet to be realized, but the promise is there. The team at Muso 'discovered' this protocol through multiple conversations with community members and their CHWs; they listened deeply and heard that time, distance, and related costs were insurmountable. They altered their protocols to accommodate this local wisdom and lived experience, and the results are exemplary. Their early experiences speaking to community members using anthropologic life history methods is outlined in a qualitative study published in *Social Science and Medicine* (Johnson et al., 2012), and a rigorous trial to further prove this approach is currently ongoing (Muso n.d.).

Working *With* CHW Colleagues; Not *Using* CHWs

Considering CHWs as 'a technology to deliver life-saving products' instead of people struggling to make a living while simultaneously improving their communities is an important error. A common turn of phrase that represents the unfortunate position in which our CHW colleagues are often placed is when health system leaders say: '*We use CHWs to* [achieve some outcome]...'. CHWs are people, not inanimate tools. To value their humanity is to begin to understand how they can be best positioned to contribute their unique inputs to complex healthcare delivery systems. Giorgio Cometto, who works at the World Health Organization and who was central in launching the new WHO guidelines on CHWs, said it succinctly:

> Do not forget that community workers are not a tool to achieve your health policy goals or a section of your policy documents or a budget line in your spreadsheet. Community workers are, first and foremost, people with families, with friends, with daily needs and difficulties, with a history rooted in their past, with a vision for their future, and especially with the right to decent working conditions and the ambition to fulfil their personal and professional dreams.

> (Cometto, 2018)

As human beings who have often lived their lives at risk of the same diseases being targeted in a health intervention they are delivering, they bring a wealth of lived experience and the wisdom that comes from a lifetime of shared challenges. This concept has been called 'what doctors cannot do', and can be the missing link for achieving new heights in health outcomes (Rosenberg, 2014).

A few examples illustrate this point well. First, we would like to highlight the work being done at the Penn CHW Center in the USA as it exemplifies many of these principles in practice, with important implications for colleagues working with CHWs in LMIC settings. The IMPaCT team (an acronym for Individualized Management for Patient-Centred Targets) have deservingly received much praise in the last few years, in part because they have achieved strong health-related outcomes within a business model that makes great sense within the often-complicated US healthcare system. Another reason is because they have studied their interventions rigorously. However, perhaps most importantly, they have demonstrated what CHWs can do when not distracted by purely 'medical tasks' when trying to improve health-related outcomes. What does it take to improve a diabetic's *average blood glucose level*? Most traditional health system programmes have turned immediately to tasks such as educating patients about the disease or encouraging patients to take their insulin. While these individual tasks are undoubtedly important, the CHWs at the Penn CHW Center are instead trusted to engage with patients in a more holistic manner and to collaboratively explore how such medical advice can be incorporated into the individuals' lives. There is no easy prescription, and solutions may range from the practical (helping someone get a copy of their birth certificate so that they can improve their insurance status) to the poetic (going bowling with someone because the last time that person felt joy was when they went bowling when younger). Critics of this approach may be quick to question the logic of such 'feel-good' interventions, but the data speaks for itself: one randomized controlled trial (RCT) found that this approach, when applied at the time of discharge from a hospitalization, improved follow-up with primary care (60% vs. 47.9%), and decreased the rates of subsequent readmissions for those patients who had already been readmitted (from 40% to 15.2%) (Kangovi et al., 2014a). Another RCT found that this approach, when applied for six months in the primary care setting, reduced hospitalizations by 65%, while increasing satisfaction scores with their care (Kangovi et al., 2018). Again, the IMPaCT team 'discovered' the secrets of their success by listening deeply to their community of patients and translating what they heard into functional protocols (Kangovi et al., 2014b).

How to Best Position CHWs

To demonstrate how CHW programmes can best incorporate the unique skills and attributes of CHWs to strengthen primary health systems in LMICs, the next section of

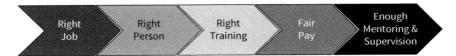

Figure 3.1 The 5-SPICE model, as five essential questions for building, evaluating, or managing a CHW programme.
Source: Adapted from Palazuelos, D., Ellis, K., DaEun Im, D. et al. 2013. 5-SPICE: The application of an original framework for community health worker program design, quality improvement and research agenda setting. *Global Health Action*, 6 (1), 19658.

this chapter provides a practical overview on how to build a CHW programme based on our experience with Partners in Health (PIH)—an NGO which has been working with CHW colleagues for nearly 30 years (Partners in Health, n.d.).

The approach utilizes a model developed by PIH and partner organizations, entitled 5-SPICE (Palazuelos, 2013). This model asks programme developers, researchers, or practitioners to consider five essential elements when creating, studying, or working to improve a CHW programme (as visualized in Figure 3.1 as five essential questions):

1) What is the *right job*, composed of the right tasks, that the CHWs need to do to achieve high-value outcomes?
2) Who is the *right person* to do those tasks?
3) What is the *best way to train them* for that job?
4) What is the *best way to motivate them* to do those tasks well, and how much payment is a *fair* amount for what is being asked?
5) How can the CHW be *best supervised and mentored*?

Right job: this is often decided by the various partners working together to develop the programme, including funders, health system stakeholders, and community beneficiaries. One way to map out how the CHW's unique contributions will support the larger health system is to consider their tasks and how they relate to the larger care cascade for that particular disorder. The Care Delivery Value Chain (CDVC) is a concept borrowed from the fields of business and management to help health system architects better plan for healthcare interventions (Kim et al. 2013). Figure 3.2 shows an example of a generic value chain, mapping out how to integrate tasks in order to generate value, which is the best possible outcome for the lowest possible cost. Box 3.1 describes an experience the first author had using the value chain to facilitate a discussion with CHWs in Guatemala about how to address the rising tide of diabetes in their communities. This example demonstrates how it is important to listen deeply to lived experiences before imposing ideas that sound good

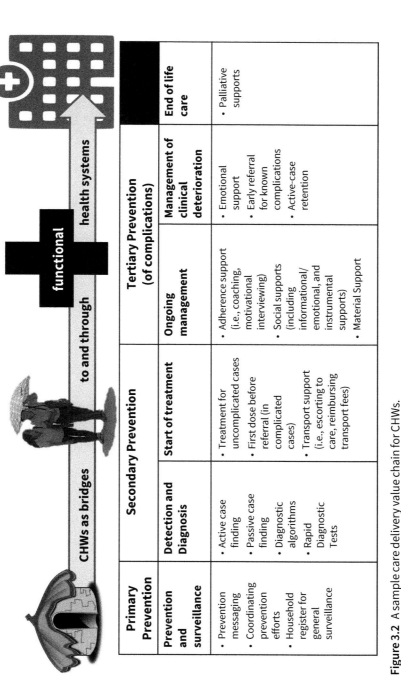

		CHWs as bridges	to and through	functional health systems	
Primary Prevention	**Secondary Prevention**			**Tertiary Prevention (of complications)**	
Prevention and surveillance	Detection and Diagnosis	Start of treatment	Ongoing management	Management of clinical deterioration	End of life care
• Prevention messaging • Coordinating prevention efforts • Household register for general surveillance	• Active case finding • Passive case finding • Diagnostic algorithms • Rapid Diagnostic Tests	• Treatment for uncomplicated cases • First dose before referral (in complicated cases) • Transport support (i.e., escorting to care, reimbursing transport fees)	• Adherence support (i.e., coaching, motivational interviewing) • Social supports (including informational/ emotional, and instrumental supports) • Material Support	• Emotional support • Early referral for known complications • Active-case retention	• Palliative supports

Figure 3.2 A sample care delivery value chain for CHWs.

Figure created using public domain images from freesvg.org, and Partners In Health Photo Archives (Community health workers—or acompañantes— Gladys Mendez and Adelaida Lopez visit patients in Chiapas, Mexico. Photo by Rebecca E. Rollins / Partners In Health)

Box 3.1   Diabetes in Guatemala, a personal experience by Dan Palazuelos, MD, MPH

In the early 2010s, I was volunteering with a small NGO in Huehuetenango, Guatemala. I was asked to train their growing cadre of volunteer CHWs about how to maintain a small medicine chest that they would manage for their communities (donated by the government of Spain). Most of the medications were what you would expect to see in a pharmacy selling relatively safe over-the-counter medications, such as antacids, mild analgesics, cough and cold medications, etc. There were, however, a few medications for hypertension and diabetes, so I became interested in how these medications could safely be included in this community-managed supply of medicines. Although there were some doctors and nurses in the area, in government hospitals and private clinics, they rarely focused on managing NCDs the way I had been trained to do in a busy primary care urban clinic in the USA; few were started on medications based on clear diagnostic criteria, and I hadn't heard of any patients getting their doses titrated based on biometric data, such as blood pressure measurements or finger stick blood glucoses. Eager to help improve the care of NCDs, but also anxious about encouraging clinical protocols that could be dangerous to patients, we started by having a facilitated debate around what made the most sense in this context. After some discussion around the need to be responsible and honest when managing a community medicine chest, I put the care delivery value chain for diabetes up on the whiteboard. The main categories present were: health promotion, making the diagnosis of diabetes, starting treatment based on that diagnosis, follow-up for ongoing care (which included the sub-tasks of maintaining the medicine chest clean and well stocked, providing treatment support for patients so that they could improve adherence to medications, and titration of medication doses based on blood glucose measurements while using an algorithm that supported decisions), and finally helping when the patient's' condition worsens (with the sub-tasks of recognizing complications, and then working on solving the problems). After they all expressed understanding of this value chain, I asked them to put a 'smiley face' next to the task that they felt most comfortable doing, and then an exclamation mark (!) next to the task they thought would be the most impactful.

It did not surprise me that all the smiley faces went next to 'health promotion' because this has always been the most common tasks assigned to CHWs all over the world. I was hoping that they would vote for 'titrating medication doses' as the most impactful intervention they could provide for the value chain. To be honest, this is because as a physician I saw this as the most important activity needed to achieve clinical control; this is the job I'm most commonly tasked to do so it must be the most important! In the fashion of 'task-shifting', I envisioned being at the forefront of a whole suite of materials, including decision-support algorithms programmed on mHealth tablets, that could aid them in achieving high levels of proficiency and safety. I was surprised when all voted for 'maintaining the medicine chest' as the most impactful task that they could focus on. When I questioned them about this, they explained that while medicine dosage titration seemed to make sense theoretically, its effect would be miniscule in a place where patients were not used to having any medications for even short periods of the year. The best dosage for them, to start, was the dose that could be given reliably without any stock outs. They were worried about taking on too medical a role, because there were already many private providers that were available to titrate medication dosages, for a price; they wanted to focus on improving reliability and dedication to continuity. It took their wisdom of the local context to teach me where to start a programme. In hindsight, this is common sense, but we are always blinded by our biases. By listening to our CHW colleagues, sometimes the obvious can finally stop being hidden in plain sight. This was nearly ten years ago when I was first starting out in my career, and the diabetes programme in Guatemala was never fully launched. My efforts ultimately transitioned to helping build another programme in Chiapas (partially with the help of at least one Guatemalan CHW who moved to Mexico to become a valued part of that team), but I carry a little piece of this early personally impactful experience in every subsequent programme with which I work.

The current enthusiasm for CHW programmes could learn a lot from this small band of Guatemalan CHWs. How many CHW programmes, developed by the best health system architects, still implement sleek training and decision-support technologies without first assuring a consistent supply chain of medications and other supplies? How many programmes assign tasks to CHWs without ever stopping to ask them what they think will be most relevant for the context?

Reproduced courtesy of Dan Palazuelos, MD, MPH.

in theory, but in practice may not be suited to the context in which they are being implemented (Figure 3.3).

Right person: this brings into question the best way to recruit and choose the best candidates and suggests that all factors be considered, from cognitive ability and the physical demands of the job, to the necessary community standing for the CHW to obtain access to the right places and people. Recruitment and selection are not simply bureaucratic steps, but rather a process that will decide whether the CHW workforce is representative and equitable. For example, many CHW programmes hold literacy as a bare minimum requirement for employment, but in many contexts, this will translate into hiring only men because women often aren't given a chance at equal schooling. If the right person doesn't exist at first, sometimes the training programme can make up the difference, that is, by including literacy training along with health service training for all socially talented but marginally literate candidates.

Right training: this will include education and training, but also a careful understanding of the skills they already possess. There are many elements to consider when formally training CHWs. Some are logistical, such as: where are they going to learn (i.e. will they have to travel, find someone to care of their children, stay the night, eat

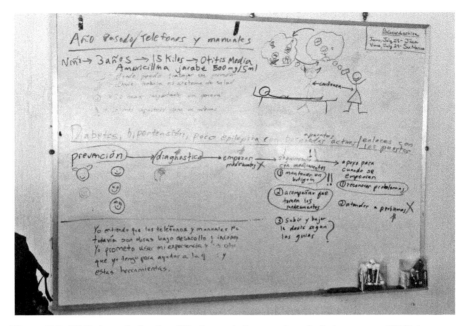

Figure 3.3 Whiteboard of a simplified care delivery value chain to engage CHWs in providing feedback on where they feel they can be most effective
Reproduced courtesy of Dan Palazuelos, MD, MPH.

meals someone else prepares)? What will be the schedule for their learning (i.e. for how many weeks, months, or years will the initial training run, and how often will new content or refresher trainings be offered)? Other elements require a deeper analysis of the context, and what the CHWs bring to their jobs even before their training starts, such as: do people in that context best learn through formal student-teacher pedagogy, traditional forms of storytelling, or perhaps even through multimedia content? Beyond the formal training process, the CHW also learns through every interaction with the health system; if doctors and nurses treat the CHWs and their patients paternalistically, there is a very real risk that the CHW will adopt that attitude. The easiest part of training a CHW is in writing and delivering a formal curriculum. The harder part is in building a health system that allows their compassion, and passion for caring, to flourish.

    <ins>Fair pay:</ins> this will include questions around whether any payment is both fair and actually enables the CHW to divert enough time away from other activities in order to focus on doing that job. The pay should be commensurate with what is being asked of the CHW, and the easiest way to assure fairness is to understand the time commitment necessary for doing the job correctly. Paying the local minimum wage for a full-time job of 40–50 hours a week is logically the right place to start. Financial payment is often considered a motivator, but in reality it is merely an enabler; payment enables a CHW to focus on their health work instead of other work

that provides for their loved ones, such as farming or selling goods. To then motivate a CHW, programme leadership should look to improving the quality of the job, as described herein.

<u>Enough mentoring or supervision:</u> how can the CHW be best supervised and mentored so that they complete tasks with excellence (meaning that they do them really well) and with fidelity (meaning that they do them really well every time)? To achieve excellence and fidelity, CHWs need to be deeply motivated, and there are many different models that have been proposed to outline all the factors that influence motivation, including the drive to acquire, bond, comprehend, and defend (i.e. the ABCD model) (Nohria et al., 2008). These elements, in turn, are most influenced by how a CHW programme is constructed and managed, and how it is situated within the larger health system and society. For the concrete task of providing oversight, we find it useful to split supportive supervision into a surveillance function (i.e. assuring a task is done as expected, such as actually going to a house to conduct a home visit), and a mentorship function (i.e. investing informational, emotional, instrumental, and material supports to help a CHW unify their desire for excellence with their ability to perform). All this will deeply influence a CHW's longevity in their job. This is an important consideration because every CHW who leaves their role prematurely represents a loss of capital costs (i.e. the funding needed to find, select, train, and mentor before they left).

The Community Health Plot Thickens

The concepts that we are proposing are not always easy to implement. To afford CHWs protected time to focus on community work instead of health work alone, and to strengthen the larger health system while building a high-impact CHW programme, significant and dedicated funding will need to secured. The benefit is that we may avoid a pitfall common to many global health failures, what has been called "the ignorance of the expert" (see Box 3.2).

The following examples help to paint a fuller picture of what is possible with such an approach and when the necessary investments are directed appropriately. Although we consider these examples successes, there are yet some elements of these programmes that are still being re-examined, tested, re-implemented, and further refined.

HIV in Liberia

Liberia is a country that has experienced incredible traumas in recent history, including a brutal civil war (1989–1997) and a debilitating Ebola epidemic (2014–2016). PIH began working in Liberia during the Ebola epidemic. However, once the epidemic had subsided, it was clear that there was still a lot of work to be done in order to help rebuild the health system. Figure 3.4 shows the number of patients enrolled in

Box 3.2 Community Wisdom in Action, an Interview with Joia Mukherjee, MD, MPH

'To me, it's the answer to the question: "How do you know you're doing the right thing [when working in global health]?" How as a foreign organization, as a white person and doctor, do I know what I am doing is correct? I know because of the community health workers, not because I think it looks right on paper. CHWs allow you to actually go to the community and see what the needs are. In that way, CHWs are the biggest defence against the ignorance of the expert.'
Joia Mukherjee, MD, MPH

When CHWs are positioned in the health system in a way that maximizes their capacity to share community wisdom, they can feel empowered to inform the 'expert' healthcare professionals. Take the following example, a story told by Dr Joia Mukherjee (Chief Medical Officer for Partners In Health). A woman is dying of cervical cancer, and unfortunately it is too late to save her life. With palliative care in mind, the medical team is trying unsuccessfully to find morphine in a resource-poor setting. What would you propose as an alternative solution? What more would you like to know about the patient and her environment in addressing this dilemma? The answer comes from a local CHW who is brought onto the care team. 'She needs a mattress, and some food.' Having visited the patient at her house, the CHW knows that she is sleeping on the bare, rocky ground and, with little access to food, she is suffering from hunger as well. The CHW's suggestion was stunningly simple yet perfectly tailored to the patients' needs. Drawing from their knowledge surrounding the reality of the patient's situation, the CHW contributed in a way that no one else on the care team could have. Therein lies the power of CHWs and what they have to offer. In the profound simplicity of their recommendations, CHWs serve as reminders that healthcare professionals are often ignorant of their patients.

In order to maximize health outcomes for the communities that they serve, health systems must train *community* health workers rather than community *health* workers. That is to say, we must avoid excessive medicalization of the role of the CHW and instead emphasize their role as community experts.

HIV care before and after the full PIH intervention was rolled out; what is evident is that enrolment, retention, and survival increased dramatically (Rogers et al. 2018).

This result was not accidental, so it is important to understand what specifically led to these outcomes. Put simply, the team focused on the three goals mapped out in the UNAIDS 90-90-90 effort: 90% of patients knowing their status, 90% being on medications, and 90% having viral load suppression. In order that more patients know their status, the health system needed to both actively screen more patients and create a clinical milieu that engendered trust. The best way to get patients to trust their health

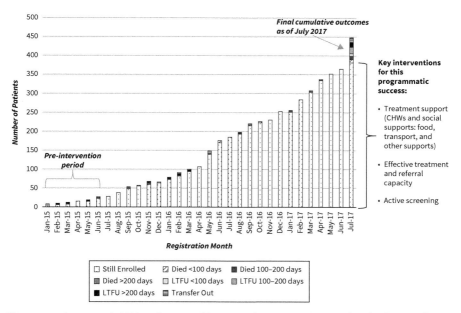

Figure 3.4 Increase in HIV patients and improved outcomes in Maryland, Liberia, after the addition of improved health system functioning, CHW-mediated treatment support, and social supports (447 patients enrolled between January 2015 and July 2017, disaggregated by month registered).

Reproduced from Rogers, J. H., Jabateh, L., Beste, J., et al. Impact of community-based adherence support on treatment outcomes for tuberculosis, leprosy and HIV/AIDS-infected individuals in post-Ebola Liberia, *Global Health Action*, 11:1, © 2018 The Authors. Distributed under the terms of the Creative Commons Attribution 4.0 International license (CC BY 4.0) (http://creativecommons.org/licenses/by/4.0/).

system is to offer quality healthcare that reaches the highest possible levels of patient-centredness, accessibility, affordability, equity, safety, and efficacy (among other metrics of quality) (Boozary et al., 2014). Indeed, when it is perceived that an HIV diagnosis represents a death sentence, it is reasonable that patients won't trust their health system; when this same diagnosis represents a chronic disease, trust may flow more freely. The PIH team in Liberia built a trustworthy health system by strengthening 'the 5 Ss': staff, stuff, spaces, systems, and social supports (see Figure 3.5).

CHWs were included in the 'staff' category, but it is important to recognize that they played an essential but *insufficient* role. Active case finding comes in many forms, including 'opt-out' HIV testing in clinics (where testing is the default option that patients can decline) or community outreach that brings testing closer to the patients' homes. These efforts help to achieve the goal of 90% of patients knowing their status. For the second goal of having 90% of patients on medications, one needs to rely on stuff (i.e. the medications), spaces (i.e. the clinics and warehouses), and systems (i.e. supply chain management preventing stock outs). For the final 90%, where patients actually achieve viral load suppression, there needs to be optimized adherence to the

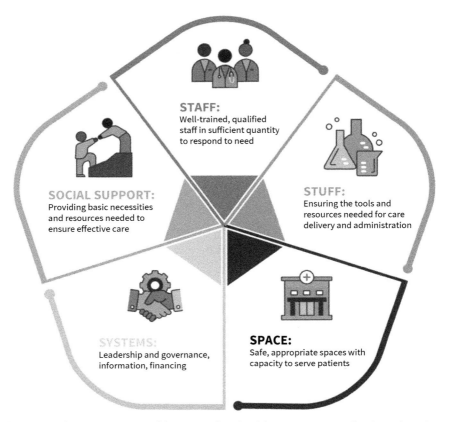

Figure 3.5 The Partners in Health approach to health systems strengthening: The 5 Ss.

medication regime and enough access to second-line medications as resistance increases. The CHWs in Liberia played an indispensable role in this final goal by extending treatment support to the patients, going to their houses, and working with them in a collaborative manner to see how they could improve their adherence to their medications.

Three components of their activities include: (1) *clinic immersion*, where there is a conscious effort to ensure that the CHWs are a part of the clinic-based team; (2) *community immersion*, where the CHWs are primarily positioned in the community to be a constant and compassionate presence; and (3) *community engagement and health promotion*, where CHWs are present in community life through the performance of dramas, radio talk shows, and door-to-door awareness. In this model, the approach is not DOT (directly observed therapy) but rather what has been called 'accompaniment', which is walking with someone, or something, through a journey.

For the patient, accompaniment means going from near death due to AIDS to viral load suppression; for the health system, accompaniment means going from an under-funded and forgotten system, to working towards achieving the 90-90-90 goals. Accompaniment is therefore both a philosophical stance and a rubric for program-matic design, and these two sides are complementary, as evident in the final 'S': social supports. In addition to a health system and CHW-mediated treatment support, the patients also had access to transport reimbursements, food packages, and additional supports on an as-needed basis. Addressing social supports may seem to some like mere charity, but in reality, it is so much more. Holistically supporting patients as they overcome barriers to effective care, often by helping to address key social determin-ants, validates their humanity; it tangibly positions the axis of their poor health not on their decisions alone but rather on the challenges they know only too well. Practically, social supports improve health outcomes and improve the return on the investment made in funding healthcare services. Although uncommon in global health, this ex-perience demonstrates how such supports are indispensable.

Overall, a key lesson from Liberia is that while CHWs should be positioned to be community-based and patient-centred, these elements alone are not enough. They also need to be supported by a larger health system that itself is robust and responsive to the ways patients actually need to live their lives. These dramatic clinical changes in Liberia may not have been possible without a combination of all of these interven-tions, working together towards the same goal.

Diabetes and Hypertension in Mexico

The future of health in many countries looks like what Mexico has been battling for the last few decades: an epidemiologic transition from infectious diseases to non-communicable diseases (NCDs) that is actually an epidemiologic overlap, a dual burden of disease. While deaths from infections like TB are decreasing, the immuno-suppressive effects of some NCDs such as diabetes remain an important risk factor for the persistence of TB in the poorest and most vulnerable (Ponce-de-Leon, 2004). In addition, the progressive damages inflicted on the bodies with chronic diseases threatens to unleash a second wave of heart, brain, kidney, and other diseases that are often considerably more expensive to treat (Stevens et al., 2008).

As such, the PIH team in Chiapas, Mexico, developed a CHW programme that would offer many of the same supports seen in other projects, and that was built around the values of accompaniment that we discussed earlier. They would improve the quality of primary care being delivered by strengthening 'the 5 Ss', and in add-ition they would ensure that CHWs extended warm, human-centred support to the patients' homes through regular home visits, emotional support, and motivational interviewing as needed. By rolling out the CHW programme in a stepped-wedge fashion, they could analyse the results in a phased manner. The 'stepped-wedge' de-sign of the analysis allows researchers the ability to position patients waiting for the intervention as a control group, and thus yields greater certainty that the intervention actually caused the changes being observed. The results from this initiative clearly show that when added to improved primary care and a consistent supply chain of medications, CHWs were able to improve clinical control for diabetes and hypertension. Specifically, there was a two-fold odds of improved clinical control (Newman et al., 2018). But despite achieving rates of clinical control rarely seen in Mexico, especially in rural Mexico or even in similar impoverished Latin American contexts, there is still not 100% clinical control of all the diseases. This has also not been achieved in any other context, including places with exemplar health systems and highly motivated patient populations such as Japan, Canada, or the Nordic countries, but the ultimate aspiration for health systems globally, including Mexico, should be absolute control of all diseases. Yet, how can this be made a reality? Figure 3.6 illustrates how much clinical control can be expected to improve for patients who get to work with CHWs, beyond the baseline control offered by strong clinic-based care. The remaining gap in achieving universal control suggests that more interventions will be necessary.

This is where the wisdom of CHWs may help to play an important role. First, their local experience already plays an incredible role in reaching each patient on an

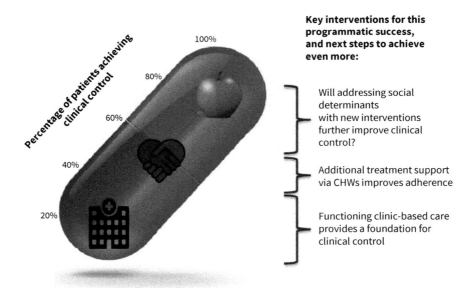

Figure 3.6 Clinic-based care lays the groundwork for clinical control of diabetes and hypertension, but CHW-mediated treatment support represents the next layer to increase the percentage of patients achieving clinical control. However, even after leveraging the expertise of CHWs, there remains room for further interventions to achieve universal control.

Figure created using public domain images from freesvg.org

individual basis during the regular home visits. Diabetes and hypertension, however, are different diseases compared to HIV and TB because the efficacy of the treatment is influenced by greater factors than the medication being used. For TB and HIV, if the pathogen is not resistant to the medication, the medication will work as long as the patient takes it as prescribed. For diabetes and hypertension, however, factors such as food quality and quantity, exercise, emotional health, and possibly genetic predisposition (amongst others) all play a major role as to whether or not efficacy will be realized. As a result, the PIH team in Mexico is currently working with CHW colleagues to jointly consider what else can be done to achieve better levels of clinical control. For example, how can communities counteract the toxicities of the processed food industry? The tobacco industry? A built environment that favours sedentary lifestyles, often in Mexico most prominently for women?

The uncomfortable truth is that many of the social determinants of these risk factors are bigger than even the best health systems can confront alone. The lesson from this experience in Mexico, therefore, shows that even the best CHW programmes are necessary but insufficient. What is needed now are new ideas, particularly when the current imagination for what is possible when building new healthcare delivery systems is proving to be insufficient in the face of our greatest global health challenges. CHWs are incredibly well positioned to offer both the creative insights to develop new protocols and the leadership to put such protocols into action, yet this will be difficult if they are only 'lackeys' doing the tasks that no one else wants to do. Our experience is that they will speak clearly, if given a chance to be heard, and will often list new food options, new transport mechanisms, better housing, and new employment opportunities as key themes. Food, transport, housing, and employment may be considered outside the purview of a traditional health delivery system, but nascent experiences in some health systems show promise that investing in this can improve outcomes and lower costs in the long run (Mozaffarian et al., 2019)

How community health workers can help improve even more 'upstream' social determinants, such as the policies that affect their health, speaks to their potentially larger role as community organizers and political activists, a topic we will explore further in the next section.

Pitfalls to Avoid

There have been projects involving CHWs that encountered barriers to success from which we can learn important lessons. Here, we highlight examples from two very well-known, large, and ultimately successful programmes in India and Ethiopia respectively. We highlight these previously published challenges not as a criticism, but to demonstrate how our colleagues working in these programmes continue to learn from their experiences and teach the rest of us how to make better decisions when building CHW programmes.

The Accredited Social Health Activist (ASHA) Programme in India

The ASHA programme (an acronym for Accredited Social Health Activist) is an Indian CHW programme that was started in 2005. By 2019, there were nearly one million female ASHAs carrying out work across India, with almost one ASHA per village (Ved et al., 2019). Their job is to connect community members to health services and to provide basic health education and medical care (such as blood pressure monitoring and identifying pregnancy complications), with a focus on encouraging women to deliver their babies in health facilities rather than at home. The ASHAs contribute to meeting certain quantitative health policy goals, including increasing immunization rates and the percentage of women receiving three or more antenatal check-ups. Box 3.3 outlines the essential elements of how the programme is structured, and Figure 3.7 shows how ASHAs are distributed across India.

Although successful by many measures, researchers undertaking qualitative work with the ASHAs have found in their analysis that at times the programme has been received with mixed feelings by the ASHAs themselves. These CHWs have expressed that they enjoy their community role and elevated social status but feel that their energies are divided and underappreciated (Scott & Shanker, 2010).

A quotation from Scott and Shanker is illustrative: 'When frontline health workers divide their energy between multiple tasks, their priorities echo the biases of the health system. There was little evidence of the critical dialogue that would be necessary to mediate between village traditions and biomedical services and begin a process of social change' (Scott & Shanker, 2010, p. 1609).

What may also be at the root of some of this discontent is the way in which ASHAs are remunerated for their efforts (Wang et al., 2012). Considered volunteers overall, they are also given performance-based compensation for specific reported activities, all of which are medical work instead of community work. This compensation varies regionally, but the analysis by Scott and Shanker quotes amounts that are similar to the compensation scheme outlined in Box 3.3. These authors hypothesize that this payment structure incentivizes the ASHAs role to become primarily medical and task-oriented; the ASHAs during this analysis earned wages only for bringing community members to the clinic and assisting with biomedical interventions, and not for promoting village health meetings or discussing more general determinants of health. Therefore, there was far less incentive for the ASHAs to leverage the full potential of their role.

Though this programme was designed with the philosophy for the ASHAs to serve as activists for broader change in health outcomes—the term 'activist' is even in their name—they have been given less space to do so (Fathima et al., 2015). Relating back to the dichotomy mentioned earlier in this chapter, of the CHW as liberator or lackey, an activist could ideally be someone who acts as a liberator, who works with community members to reflect on the root causes of their illnesses and then combines joint action

Box 3.3 Training and Responsibilities of ASHAs

Recruitment

- ASHAs must be female, between 21 and 45 years old with middle-school education (class eight or higher), and ideally should be a 'daughter-in-law' of the village, either married, widowed, or divorced with a likelihood to live in the village for the foreseeable future.
- States have flexibility in selecting ASHAs with lower literacy levels to ensure adequate community representation and local residence.

Training

- The ASHAs receive training supported by the Government of India for 23 days spread over 12 months. Training models may vary by state and may involve partnerships with various NGOs and other training centers.
- The ASHAs are expected to attend periodic review meetings and ongoing job training (12 additional days per year).

Primary Responsibilities

- Expected to work about 2.3 hours per day and 4 days per week, except during events such as training and immunization days.
- Create awareness and provide information to the community on the determinants of health such as nutrition, basic sanitation and hygiene, and existing health services.
- Counsel mothers on birth preparedness, safe delivery, feeding practices, immunization, prevention of common infections, and family planning
- Registering all pregnant women, provide three antenatal visits and two postnatal visits, and facilitate access to health services for the mother and child.
- Rollout of other government programmes such as the *Janani Surakshna Yojana* (JSY)—a cash entitlement programme to incentivize women to give birth in health facilities.
- Arrange escort or accompany pregnant women and children requiring treatment to health facilities.
- Additional responsibilities of the ASHAs may vary by state.
- Act as a bridge between the rural population and the government health system.

Compensation

- The ASHAs are honorary volunteers and receive performance-based compensation based on reported activities.

- The compensation varies by the state and by the type of services provided. It ranges from INR 200 (~$2.95) for registering a pregnant woman, providing three antenatal and two postnatal visits to INR 200–350 (~$2.95–5) for facilitating institutional birth.

Supervision
- As per national guidelines, one ASHA facilitator is assigned for every 20 ASHAs, to help with selection, provide on-the-job mentoring, conduct regular supervisory meetings, and maintain records.
- During monthly performance monitoring meetings, ASHAs are to report on their activities, especially around critical tasks around visiting newborns on the first day for home deliveries, attending immunization camps, visiting households to discuss nutrition, and acting as DOT providers for tuberculosis treatment.

to address those issues. Interviews with ASHAs illuminated that they are not aware of what it means or entails to serve as activists, and their training pays little attention to developing their skills in such a role (Saprii et al., 2015). By paying for more easily measurable medical tasks and services, this programme is reproducing a trend common in other health systems, such as the 'fee-for-service' reimbursement schedule in the USA that favours interventions and procedures over counselling and primary care; in both cases the system gets more of what it pays for. The ASHA programme is certainly one of the largest and most successful CHW programmes globally, and the efforts of the ASHAs have been associated with improved maternal-child health behaviours. We offer these insights to illustrate how a pay-for-performance scheme can incentivize CHWs to focus on some tasks over others, but that this can have unintended consequences as they struggle to balance what they are paid to do versus other activities.

On the other hand, what would be the best ways to incentivize CHWs to direct their focus on activities such as illness prevention, environmental rights, water rights, village mobilization for health action, improving nutrition, etc.? As we saw with the Mexico case above, these actions could arguably have the greatest impact, but the road to that impact is not clear and may be difficult to travel. This could be one of the most exciting frontiers for future CHW programmes to explore.

Health Extension Workers and Integrated Community Case Management in Ethiopia

In 2004, Ethiopia started the national Health Extension Programme in an effort to achieve Millennium Development Goal 4 (MDG 4—to reduce under-five mortality

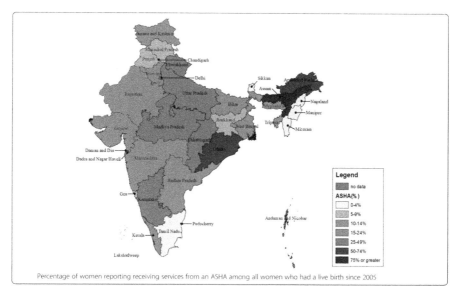

Percentage of women reporting receiving services from an ASHA among all women who had a live birth since 2005

Figure 3.7   Percentage of women reporting receiving services from an ASHA among all women who had a live birth since 2005.

Reproduced from Agarwal, S., Curtis, S.L., Angeles, G., et al. The impact of India's accredited social health activist (ASHA) program on the utilization of maternity services: A nationally representative longitudinal modelling study. *Human resources for health*, 17 (1), 68. © 2019 The Authors. Distributed under the terms of the Creative Commons Attribution 4.0 International License (CC BY 4.0) (http://creativecommons.org/licenses/by/4.0/).

by two-thirds). A key component of this programme was to train 30,000 health extension workers (HEWs) to provide and encourage the use of preventive care and some healthcare treatments. From 2004 to 2009, HEWs were trained in the iCCM protocol, which includes treating diarrhoea with oral rehydration therapy (ORT), malaria with artemisinin-based combination therapy (ACT) after a positive rapid diagnostic test, and severe acute undernutrition with ready-to-use therapeutic foods (RUTF). In 2009, the iCCM model was broadened to include treatment of uncomplicated pneumonia with antibiotics. HEWs also promoted health education centred around 16 key messages and worked to identify major life events such as births, deaths, and pregnancies (Amouzou et al., 2016).

However, despite all their training and support, including receiving a community-built clinic to work in and a good stock of supplies, a study by Amouzou and colleagues found that the HEWs were not able to reduce under-five mortality (ibid.). It was a low utilization of services that weakened the programme; mothers simply did not bring their children to the new clinic with the new type of health worker (in fact, only 8.5% of children 2–59 months old with fever sought or got care from a HEW). *Why* this happened highlights an important lesson for the future of CHWs everywhere, not only Ethiopia.

First, this programme should be credited for several strengths. The iCCM programme was designed well and implemented rapidly, yet effectively. The programme also benefitted from effective and clinically focused training, appropriate supervision, and high-quality training materials and job aids (Nsibande et al., 2018). At the same time, the implementation of certain skills was lacking; for example only one-third of severe cases with any of the targeted diseases received proper management, and only half of such cases that required referrals actually received one. Amouzou and colleagues outlined five reasons for low utilization (Amouzou et al., 2013). Two were the effects of geography and social networks, but we want to highlight the three other reasons in particular as we believe they are central to why the CHWs in this context were initially unable to achieve maximum impact:

1. *Negative perceptions of quality:* community acceptance of the HEWs was a major barrier to utilization because of the perception that HEWs provided low-quality services, lacked sensitivity to community needs, and neglected certain villages and populations. Communities likely saw them as providers of low-quality care, influenced by their experience with CHWs prior to the iCCM training programme, and possibly also because HEWs were often absent from health posts. A related lesson is that CHW programmes should be built for success, and the coverage ratios at this point were quite high: 2 CHWs per 5000 people spread out over a large geographic area. It is very difficult to achieve high coverage, ensure geographic accessibility, or implement an active and equitable coverage with ratios like this.

2. *A mismatch between supply quality and demand:* the design of the iCCM programme improved the supply of healthcare services, but it paid less attention to the quality of that supply, and to other activities that could generate demand for those services. Although it was up to the HEWs to raise awareness of their position and services among key informants, such as community and religious leaders, and to inform parents to take their sick children to health posts, they were also busy with their primary responsibility of providing care in the community. Patients already had a negative perception of the type of care that could be provided by CHWs, based on historical experiences, so despite the efforts to improve this situation there was insufficient dialogue to understand and negotiate a new space at this intersection between quality and the perception of quality.

3. *Outside recruitment:* a majority of HEWs were not recruited from the communities they were serving, making them outsiders or newcomers to their patients. This further impeded the dialogue that needed to take place, and the social capital that needed to be amassed to improve knowledge about, and acceptance of, this new programme. Locals naturally know their community best, and this lived experience can facilitate a deeper entry point for impactful community health work.

When reviewing these challenges faced by the iCCM programme, critical lessons surface. When a programme is centrally planned, without community input, barriers to its overall acceptance may appear and potentially jeopardize the overall success of the programme. The key lesson from this case study is the need to include the community voice from the earliest possible stage in design and implementation, in order to ensure the programme is responsive to their needs and begins to generate trust in the services it provides. Trust is complex but essential in a community health programme. Key dimensions of trust identified in one qualitative study included: 'perceived competence, assurance of treatment irrespective of ability to pay or at any time of the day, patients' willingness to accept drawbacks in healthcare, loyalty to the provider and respect for the provider' (Gopichandran & Chetlapalli, 2013). Only some of these dimensions were met, and the CHWs themselves suffered as a result.

Since identification of these challenges, rather than shy away from them, the Ethiopian government has tried to learn from this experience and respond in constructive ways. One such response was to assemble and deploy a health development army (HDA), a volunteer cadre designed to help bridge some of the gaps mentioned above (Kok et al., 2015). The HEW model had been designed around a largely medical model; however, the HDA model incorporated a great level of community engagement. The more time that the HDA CHWs have to focus on their patients, the better the results are. One study found that when reducing the ratios of houses assigned to each HDA, from more than 60 per HDA to 40, there was higher coverage of antenatal care, institutional deliveries, clean cord care, and thermal care (Betemariam et al., 2017). Reducing ratios and allowing the CHWs more time to approach assigned tasks better will require more CHWs to cover the same population, which in turn requires a larger budget to train and manage that workforce, but this is a worthwhile investment; community work can improve the results of health work, but only if CHWs are invested in and supported accordingly.

Women's Development Groups (WDGs) have also been instituted to identify pregnant women and to work with HEWs to refer them to health facilities via ambulance when needed. This has led to an increase in the rates of skilled birth attendance in some regions (Jackson et al., 2016), thereby demonstrating how a combination of community voice, health system coordination, and new investments (i.e. ambulances to address transportation barriers) can be effective. Utilization of health facilities for births has also been improved by providing culturally accountable and respectful services (Jackson & Hailemariam, 2016). And an analysis in 2015 found that there had been a statistically significant upward trend in delivery care and postnatal care in all types of facilities in Northern Ethiopia from 2002 to 2012 (Gebrehiwot et al., 2015), suggesting that the health extension programme had been able to leverage the lessons learned from its initial challenges to yield opportunities for growth and improved outcomes.

Among many, the lessons from Ethiopia show how the outcomes of health systems can be improved if there are mechanisms to activate and incorporate insights from the community and CHWS, if care providers then adapt their practices to these inputs, and the health system strategically increases the investments necessary to improve the delivery of quality care. Good quality care, dialogue, respect, and accountability are reproducible mechanisms for improving trust, and trust is indispensable for achieving health-related impacts.

Summary and Future Horizons

Our central hypothesis in this chapter is that community health workers are capable of contributing otherwise unavailable functionality to health systems if they are both allowed and empowered to do so. To 'allow them' means to give them the space to do what they do best: be in their community physically and interact with other community members so that they are best positioned to know the details and wisdom that only that position and experience will allow. To 'empower them' means to give them all the elements necessary to work effectively (i.e. fair compensation for their time, other financial protections, robust training, appropriate supervision and mentorship so that they perform their tasks with excellence and fidelity, etc.).

The future of community health will be brightest when all CHWs themselves see their work as a long-term vocation. If it remains common that they aspire to become nurses, doctors, or other common care providers, then this means that their job is too medicalized, micromanaged, and under-resourced to truly consider them a member of the healthcare delivery team. Perhaps we should gauge success by how many doctors and nurses want to become community health workers instead? While CHWs should always have the ability to choose their career paths, it is up to the larger global health delivery community to assure those choices include this vision. CHWs can only be as strong as the systems supporting them. If they fail, it is because we have failed them.

References

Amouzou, A., Hazel, E., Shaw, B., Miller, N.P., Tafesse, M., Mekonnen, Y., et al. (2016). Effects of the integrated community case management of childhood illness strategy on child mortality in Ethiopia: A cluster randomized trial. *American Journal of Tropical Medicine and Hygiene*, 94(3), 596–604.

Betemariam, W., Damtew, Z., Tesfaye, C., Fesseha, N., & Karim, A.M. (2017). Effect of Ethiopia's health development army on maternal and newborn health care practices: A multi-level cross-sectional analysis. *Annals of Global Health*, 83(1), 24.

Boozary, A.S., Farmer, P.E., & Jha, A.K. (2014). The Ebola outbreak, fragile health systems, and quality as a cure. *Journal of American Medical Association*, 312(18), 1859–1860.

Cometto, G., 2018. Section 2: Making The Case; Evidence Based Arguments for Community Health Worker Programmes. HarvardX CHA01—Strengthening Community Health Worker Programmes. Accessed from: https://courses.edx.org/courses/course-v1:HarvardX+CHA01+2T2019/course/

Farmer, P.E., Nutt, C.T., Wagner, C.M., Sekabaraga, C., Nuthulaganti, T., Weigel, J.L., et al. (2013). Reduced premature mortality in Rwanda: Lessons from success. *British Medical Journal*, 346, f65.

Fathima, F.N., Raju, M., Varadharajan, K.S., Krishnamurthy, A., Ananthkumar, S.R., & Mony, P.K. (2015). Assessment of 'accredited social health activists'—a national community health volunteer scheme in Karnataka State, India. *Journal of Health, Population, and Nutrition*, 3(1), 137.

Freire, P. (2018). *Pedagogy of the Oppressed*. New York, Bloomsbury Publishing.

Gebrehiwot, T.G., San Sebastian, M., Edin, K., & Goicolea, I. (2015). The health extension programme and its association with change in utilization of selected maternal health services in Tigray Region, Ethiopia: A segmented linear regression analysis. *PloS ONE*, 10(7).

Gopichandran, V. & Chetlapalli, S.K. (2013). Dimensions and determinants of trust in health care in resource poor settings—a qualitative exploration. *PLoS ONE*, 8(7).

Jackson, R. & Hailemariam, A. (2016). The role of health extension workers in linking pregnant women with health facilities for delivery in rural and pastoralist areas of Ethiopia. *Ethiopian Journal of Health Sciences*, 26(5), 471–478.

Jackson, R., Tesfay, F.H., Godefay, H., & Gebrehiwot, T.G. (2016). Health extension workers' and mothers' attitudes to maternal health service utilization and acceptance in Adwa Woreda, Tigray Region, Ethiopia. *PLoS ONE*, 11(3).

Johnson, A., Goss, A., Beckerman, J., & Castro, A. (2012). Hidden costs: The direct and indirect impact of user fees on access to malaria treatment and primary care in Mali. *Social Science & Medicine*, 75(10), 1786–1792.

Johnson, A.D., Thiero, O., Whidden, C., Poudiougou, B., Diakité, D., Traoré, F., et al. (2018). Proactive community case management and child survival in periurban Mali. *British Medical Journal Global Health*, 3(2), e000634.

Kangovi, S., Mitra, N., Grande, D., White, M.L., McCollum, S., Sellman, J., et al. (2014a). Patient-centered community health worker intervention to improve posthospital outcomes: A randomized clinical trial. *Journal of American Medical Association Internal Medicine*, 17(4), 535–543.

Kangovi, S., Grande, D., Carter, T., Barg, F.K., Rogers, M., Glanz, K., et al. (2014b). The use of participatory action research to design a patient-centered community health worker care transitions intervention. *Healthcare*, 2(2), 136–144.

Kangovi, S., Mitra, N., Norton, L., Harte, R., Zhao, X., Carter, T., et al. (2018). Effect of community health worker support on clinical outcomes of low-income patients across primary care facilities: A randomized clinical trial. *Journal of American Medical Association Internal Medicine*, 178(12), 1635–1643.

Kim, J.Y., Farmer, P., & Porter, M.E. (2013). Redefining global health-care delivery. *Lancet*, 382(9897), 1060–1069.

Kok, M.C., Kea, A.Z., Datiko, D.G., Broerse, J., Dieleman, M., Taegtmeyer, M., et al. (2015). A qualitative assessment of health extension workers' relationships with the community and health sector in Ethiopia: Opportunities for enhancing maternal health performance. *Human Resources for Health*, 13(1), 80.

Mozaffarian, D., Mande, J., & Micha, R. (2019). Food is medicine—the promise and challenges of integrating food and nutrition into health care. *Journal of American Medical Association Internal Medicine*, 179(6), 793–795.

Muso (n.d.) *Muso Health*. Available from: http://www.musohealth.org/

Newman, P.M., Franke, M.F., Arrieta, J., Carrasco, H., Elliott, P., et al. (2018). Community health workers improve disease control and medication adherence among patients with diabetes and/or hypertension in Chiapas, Mexico: An observational stepped-wedge study. *British Medical Journal Global Health*, 3(1), e000566.

Nohria, N., Groysberg, B., & Lee, L. (2008). Employee motivation: A powerful new model. *Harvard Business Review*, 86(7/8), 78.

Nsibande, D., Loveday, M., Daniels, K., Sanders, D., Doherty, T., & Zembe, W. (2018). Approaches and strategies used in the training and supervision of Health Extension Workers (HEWs) delivering integrated community case management (iCCM) of childhood illness in Ethiopia: A qualitative rapid appraisal. *African Health Sciences*, 18(1), 188–197.

Palazuelos, D., Ellis, K., DaEun Im, D., Peckarsky, M., Schwarz, D., Bertrand Farmer, D., et al. (2013). 5-SPICE: The application of an original framework for community health worker programme design, quality improvement and research agenda setting. *Global Health Action*, 6(1), 19658.

Partners in Health (n.d.) *Partners in Health*. Available from: www.pih.org.

Partners In Health Report (2018). *Achieving Universal Health Coverage. Practical Strategies for the Progressive Realization of the Right to Health*. Partners In Health, Boston, MA.

Ponce-de-Leon, A., de Lourdes Garcia-Garcia, M., Garcia-Sancho, M.C., Gomez-Perez, F.J., Valdespino-Gomez, J.L., Olaiz-Fernandez, G., et al. (2004). Tuberculosis and diabetes in southern Mexico. *Diabetes Care*, 27(7), 1584–1590.

Rogers, J.H., Jabateh, L., Beste, J., Wagenaar, B.H., McBain, R., Palazuelos, D., et al. (2018). Impact of community-based adherence support on treatment outcomes for tuberculosis, leprosy and HIV/AIDS-infected individuals in post-Ebola Liberia. *Global Health Action*, 11(1), 1522150.

Rosenberg, T. (2014). What doctors cannot do. *New York Times*, Opinionator pages; 28 Aug. Available from: https://opinionator.blogs.nytimes.com/2014/08/28/what-doctors-cant-do/

Sadruddin, S., Pagnoni, F., & Baugh, G. (2019). Lessons from the integrated community case management (iCCM) Rapid Access Expansion Program. *Journal of Global Health*, 9(2).

Saprii, L., Richards, E., Kokho, P., & Theobald, S. (2015). Community health workers in rural India: Analysing the opportunities and challenges Accredited Social Health Activists (ASHAs) face in realising their multiple roles. *Human Resources for Health*, 1(1), 95.

Schneider, H. & Maleka, N. (2018). Patterns of authorship on community health workers in low-and-middle-income countries: An analysis of publications (2012–2016). *British Medical Journal Global Health*, 3(3), e000797.

Scott, K. & Shanker, S. (2010). Tying their hands? Institutional obstacles to the success of the ASHA community health worker programme in rural north India. *AIDS Care*, 2(suppl. 2), 1606–1612.

Scott, K., Beckham, S.W., Gross, M., Pariyo, G., Rao, K.D., Cometto, G., et al. (2018). What do we know about community-based health worker programmes? A systematic review of existing reviews on community health workers. *Human Resources for Health*, 16(1), 39.

Stevens, G., Dias, R.H., Thomas, K.J., Rivera, J.A., Carvalho, N., Barquera, S., et al. (2008). Characterizing the epidemiological transition in Mexico: National and subnational burden of diseases, injuries, and risk factors. *PLoS Medicine*, 5(6).

Ved, R., Scott, K., Gupta, G., Ummer, O., Singh, S., Srivastava, A., et al. (2019). How are gender inequalities facing India's one million ASHAs being addressed? Policy origins and adaptations for the world's largest all-female community health worker programme. *Human Resources for Health*, 1 (1), 3.

Wang, H., Juyal, R.K., Miner, S.A., & Fischer, E. (2012). *Performance-Based Payment System for Ashas in India: What Does International Experience Tell Us?* Bethesda, MD, The Vistaar Project, IntraHealth International Inc., Abt Associates Inc.

Werner, D., Thuman, C., Maxwell, J., Pearson, A., & Cary, F. (1993). *Where There is no Doctor: A Village Health Care Handbook for Africa*. London, Macmillan.

4

Approaches to Community Health Worker Training and Supervision

James O'Donovan

Background

The purpose of this chapter is to help position readers to understand the deep-rooted complexities surrounding community health worker (CHW) training and supervision.

It is estimated there will be a global shortage of 18 million health workers by 2030, which is more than twice the seven million shortfall estimated in 2013 (Limb, 2016). This vast scarcity of health workers will disproportionally affect countries classed as low and middle-income (LMIC), which will have a major impact in achieving the United Nations (UN) Sustainable Development Goal (SDG) 3—'Good Health and Wellbeing for All'.

One proposed solution to address the gap in human resources for health has been to consider alternative health service delivery models, which utilize lower-skilled cadres of workers. Commonly referred to as 'task shifting', this process involves re-distribution of certain healthcare related tasks away from highly qualified health professionals, such as doctors or nurses, to health workers with fewer qualifications and less training. One particular cadre that has been deployed in such a manner are CHWs.

If CHWs are properly supported, they can help to ensure health equity, save lives, increase access to care, and generate returns on investment. Yet, as history has already demonstrated, CHW programmes face multiple and complex challenges given that they are complex entities themselves, operating at the interface of the formal health system and the community, and involve multiple actors, including non-governmental organizations (NGOs), government, community, and health facility staff (Schneider, 2019). These complexities and challenges will be discussed in the next section of this chapter.

James O'Donovan, *Approaches to Community Health Worker Training and Supervision* In: *Training for Community Health.*
Edited by: Anne Geniets, James O'Donovan, Laura Hakimi, and Niall Winters, Oxford University Press.
© Oxford University Press 2021. DOI: 10.1093/oso/9780198866244.003.0004

Challenges Facing Modern CHW Programmes

CHWs are embedded within complex health systems, which involve 'large numbers of diverse elements, that interact dynamically, often in non-linear ways, informed by direct and indirect feedback, in open systems' (George et al., 2018, p. 2). Programmes are administered and monitored through a wide range of actors, ranging from official government programmes, to NGOs. This variable nature of CHW programme delivery has resulted in a patchwork landscape which is difficult to navigate and regulate, both by the health workers, members of the community seeking care, and local governance. For example, in Mozambique it has been estimated that over 90% of The President's Emergency Plan for AIDS Relief (PEPFAR) funding flows 'off-budget' to NGO 'implementing partners', with little left for the public health system (Pfeiffer & Chapman, 2019). In one instance, CHWs in Mozambique (who are referred to as *Activistas* or *Agentes Polivalentes Elementares* (APEs)) received funding from three different NGOs to support the delivery of HIV and maternal and child health services. This resulted in confusion between the facility based nurses who did not know which NGOs the Activistas were working for (Pfeiffer & Chapman, 2019).

Furthermore, many programmes have been criticized for being too narrow in focus and taking a 'vertical approach' towards implementation (Simon et al., 2009), meaning they often focus on one particular disease or system; for example some CHWs are trained only to manage maternal or children health issues, whereas others are trained only to manage ear disease. By taking this siloed approach, programmes fail to capture the complexity of the systems within which CHWs are embedded, as well as how they might contribute to wider health system strengthening (Palazuelos et al., 2018). High rates of attrition are prevalent, especially in models where CHWs are volunteers (vs. paid). In addition, CHWs often face inadequate working conditions and lack support to fulfil the tasks expected of them. This includes infrequent, poorly structured training and a lack of supervision.

In this context, training refers to the initial period of sensitization and formal education of CHWs across a range of topics, including those specific to particular areas of disease they are expected to manage (such as the recognition, prevention, and treatment of malaria). In contrast, supervision refers to the process of supporting the CHWs in an ongoing and continuous fashion to ensure they remain up to date, competent, and are appropriately supported and mentored in their job roles.

This chapter will provide a brief history of training and supervision in relation to the wider field of healthcare more generally, followed by an overview of the current state of CHW training and supervision. This will include highlighting some of the key barriers and opportunities facing CHW training. The chapter will conclude by suggesting areas for future work, which will be expanded upon in subsequent chapters.

A Brief History of Training and Supervision in Healthcare

The primary function of training healthcare professionals has traditionally been viewed as a way to enhance their knowledge and skills in order to improve patient care. This has often led to the prioritization of these aspects over and above other purposes of training, such as holistic features of professional development as an individual. Subsequently, the purpose of health worker training, especially in the context of CHWs, has failed to acknowledge and address the need to facilitate autonomous learners, working in a supportive environment to assist both professional *and* personal growth. This can perhaps be explained by the broader historical context of health worker training and supervision.

Formal training (e.g. classroom based lectures led by an instructor and 'delivered' to students) and supervision in healthcare has its roots in organizational and management processes that can be traced back to the early 1900s. In 1904, Jeffrey Brackett outlined the role of supervision in social work in his book *Supervision and Education in Charity* (Kadushin & Harkness, 2014). Brackett stated that the purpose of training and supervision was to 'help the social worker develop practice, knowledge and skills, and provide emotional support to the person in the social work role' (Kadushin & Harkness, 2014, p. 1). Yet, as Bernard and Goodyear (1992) note, the interpretation of what training and supervision should entail changed over time, so that by the end of the 1900s the field of healthcare appeared to prioritize administrative functions over supportive ones. They suggested that more emphasis was placed on accountability than emotional support, with hierarchy and evaluation deeply intertwined within this. This style of training and supervision, which is more controlling in nature, often places emphasis on fault finding. There is often a unidirectional flow of information, where the trainer or supervisor assumes the role of the expert, whose job is to 'transmit the knowledge they possess' to the individual being trained or supervised.

Recognizing that this style of training and supervision fails to motivate health workers (Crigler et al., 2013), efforts have been made over the past decade to shift towards a model which places greater emphasis on the needs of health workers as learners. The ideals of this model are to promote collaborative problem solving, where the exchange of ideas and information is more reciprocal in nature (Tavrow et al., 2002; Clements et al., 2007; Hill et al., 2014). In the case of health worker training, in recent years there has been an epistemological shift away from pedagogical models of information dissemination, towards ones which focus on collaborative problem solving that are underpinned by social constructivism, such as problem based learning. Such models have proven to be particularly popular in the training of medical students, and several universities around the world now advocate for this style of learning. Similarly, in the case of supervision, it is widely accepted that 'supportive supervision' is the ideal model by which to support health workers. The WHO defines supportive supervision as:

A process of helping staff to improve their own work performance continuously. It is carried out in a respectful and non-authoritarian way with a focus on using supervisory visits as an opportunity to improve knowledge and skills of health staff. Supportive supervision encourages open two-way communication, and building team approaches that facilitate problem-solving. It focuses on monitoring performance towards goals, and using data for decision-making, and depends upon regular follow-up with staff to ensure that new tasks are being implemented correctly.

(World Health Organization, 2008)

Significantly, in a landmark study by Roberton et al. (2015), a call was made to re-define how supervision was delivered, by focusing less on 'report checking and more on problem solving and skills development' (Roberton et al., 2015, p. 1).

At this point, it is important to note that considering CHWs as an extension of the formal medical system runs the risk of not fully understanding or appreciating their unique position within society. For example, unlike other cadres of professional health workers, one of the key attributes of a CHW is that they are selected from their own communities in which they live and work. Second, the expectations community members have of them are different to formal professionals. While they are expected to play a role in healthcare delivery, they are also likely to play a greater role in community advocacy and emotional support. Thus, by taking an approach to training and supervision which prioritizes knowledge and skills acquisition over other important aspects of their job, such as trust and respect, there is a danger that current practices fail to acknowledge the holistic role CHWs play within their communities. Training and supervisory programmes should therefore be designed and delivered in a contextually and culturally appropriate manner, in order that they contribute to the supportive environment necessary for CHWs to flourish, and contribute towards health system strengthening.

However, the concept of what good training and supervision *actually* means to front-line health workers, and how it should be delivered and evaluated in practice remains underexplored. It is only more recently that attempts have been made to try and conceptualize how good training supervision should be structured. These will be discussed in the next section.

What Are Key Aspects of 'Good' Training and Supervision?

Across the field of medical education attempts have been made at trying to conceptualize 'effective training and supervision', and in an article by Kilminster et al. (2007), seven features were identified. These principles state that training and supervision should be:

1. Offered in context.
2. Direct and respectful, including positive exchanges between supervisors and supervisees.
3. Provide frequent constructive and focused feedback.
4. Structured and offered regularly. Content, duration, and number of meetings should be agreed in advance to set realistic expectations.
5. Holistic and encompass 'clinical management; teaching and research; management and administration; pastoral care; interpersonal skills; personal development; reflection'.
6. Led by the needs of the health worker and involve a reflective process.
7. Ensure those responsible for training and supervision receive training on 'understanding teaching; assessment; counselling skills; appraisal; feedback; careers advice; interpersonal skills' (Kilminster et al., 2007, p. 2).

In addition to these seven features, it was also deemed important that those in charge of training and supervision should be able to demonstrate an element of clinical competence. This is because one of the core priorities in healthcare is that of 'patient safety and the quality of patient care' (Tomlinson, 2015, p. 7).

Specific to CHWs, Duthie et al. (2012) outlined key features of effective training and supervision, including advocating for CHWs, thoughtful recruitment, developing field sensitivity, respecting and trusting the CHW, clarifying boundaries and scope of practice, developing a flexible structure, and encouraging continuous learning. Crucially, although there are many parallels between the two sets of recommendations, there are also some key differences. For example, the recommendations put forward by Duthie et al. (2012) place greater emphasis on respecting the cultural contexts in which CHWs operate. In addition they recognize how CHWs have different needs and responsibilities to other healthcare professionals, since they need to 'be able to relate to community members in a way that is often not possible for health professionals who have different cultural or socioeconomic background(s)' (Duthie et al., 2012, p. 63).

Yet, despite these attempts to try and define and conceptualize effective supervision, little empirical work has been done to explore how these features can be achieved in practice with front-line health workers (Hernández et al., 2014). The next section will therefore outline the current landscape and existing work with regards to CHW training and supervision.

Training and Supervision of CHWs in LMICs

In 2018, a comprehensive report was published by six leading NGOs responsible for developing high-impact CHW programmes with governments and communities across the world. Eight features were outlined in the report, describing the 'minimum viable elements needed for CHW programmes to succeed' (Ballard et al., 2018, p. 25). These included the need for CHWs to be accredited, accessible, proactive, continuously trained, supported by a dedicated supervisor, financially remunerated, a member of the formal health system, and part of continuous data feedback loops (Cometto et al., 2018). The importance placed on training and supervision in this report mirrors the findings of other studies, which conclude that high quality training, and ongoing supervision are key features of strong CHW programmes, resulting in improved CHW performance, motivation, retention, and job satisfaction.

However, despite these claims around the importance of training and supervision, they remain one of the most under-researched areas of CHW programming to date. CHW training programmes are often disjointed, one-off events, with the existing literature containing poor descriptions of how training programmes are designed.

For example, a 2013 report commissioned by the One Million Community Health Worker Campaign, which aimed to understand current practices in CHW training in sub-Saharan Africa and South Asia found a 'significant lack of formal research on CHW training' (One Million CHWs, 2014). Of the work that exists, much of it is fraught with challenges, including 'a lack of in-service training; lack of adaption to support local languages; inconsistent delivery methods, irregular and insufficient monitoring and evaluation practices; lack of coordination with other service providers; lack of emphasis on communication skills; and an overuse of rote techniques' (One Million CHWs, 2014). Similarly, Leslie et al. (2016), described the quality of evidence regarding the effects of supervision as 'weak', and that 'the magnitude and longevity of the effect on provider quality has not been definitively established' (Leslie et al., 2016, p. 1717).

The first issue it that the existing empirical literature often fails to define the purpose of CHW training and supervision. This means that the current landscape of research on CHW training and supervision lacks clarity and coherence. There is no 'golden thread' running through the field; in part due to the disparate number of actors each staking a claim to CHW training across multiple geographical contexts. As such, leading scholars in the field such as Hill et al. (2014), have called for future work to better define and frame the field of CHW training and supervision (Hill et al., 2014). This includes the need for work to provide clear descriptions of the purpose of training, and type of supervision that is taking place. This includes programme components and processes. Given the disjointed nature of the field, it is also imperative that descriptions of training and supervision programmes position their work with regards to ongoing initiatives. This will help those working in the field to better understand best practices, and how new initiatives link to existing ones.

Second, despite claims being made in the existing literature around the benefits of training and supervision, it is not clear as to what these benefits are, whom they serve, and the mechanisms by which they occur. One of the first comprehensive systematic reviews regarding training and supervision for primary health workers in LMIC settings was published in 2014 (Bosch-Capblanch & Marceau, 2014). The authors of this study noted that the purpose and focus of training and supervision was largely centred around administrative aspects (Bosch-Capblanch & Marceau, 2014), rather than a focus on problem solving, clinical supervision, training and consultation with the community. From a participatory standpoint, this positioning of training and supervision is problematic, since by over emphasizing the administrative purposes of training and supervision, other more holistic aspects are in danger of being overlooked.

A second review by Hill et al. (2014) noted that between the early 2000s and late 2010s there was a shift in focus away from viewing supervision as a management tool, towards one where supervision was regarded as a way to address the needs of CHWs as learners (Hill et al., 2014). The review also highlighted that although supervision strategies that were supportive and encouraged community engagement showed promise, the evaluation of such programmes was weak. Hill et al. (2014) also noted that CHWs and CHW supervisors are not 'blank pages' (Hill et al., 2014). Their perceptions of supervision will inevitably be influenced by existing values and previous experience (Hill et al., 2014).

Working alongside CHWs is therefore of paramount importance so that these values can be appropriately incorporated in the development of training and supervisory programmes. It is noticeable that the current field of CHW training and education seemingly fails to acknowledge such perspectives, with many programmes being designed by taking a top-down approach. Those responsible for designing CHW training and supervision programmes must therefore seek to develop epistemological world awareness when designing supervisory and training programmes, which can be modified and adapted to the constantly changing experiences of CHWs. Taking more participatory approaches towards the design of CHW training and supervision could therefore represent one potential opportunity.

It is also worth documenting and acknowledging some of the specific challenges faced in the delivery of CHW training and supervision, so that those responsible for programme delivery can attempt to address such challenges from the outset. These challenges, although not exhaustive, will be outlined in the next section.

Challenges Surrounding Training and Supervision of CHWs in LMICs

In order for training and supervision to occur, an enabling environment has to be in place. However, this is often difficult due to several barriers and challenges. These include, but are not limited to: human resource shortages; challenges related to trainers and supervisors; disjointed supervisory and training frameworks; infrastructure barriers; competing interests; and funding challenges.

Human-Resource Shortages

A lack of human resources for health has resulted in a shortage of CHW trainers and supervisors in many LMICs. This means that trainer: trainee ratios are often unacceptably high, which has been suggested to affect the overall quality of training and supervision (Rosales et al., 2015). It is also important to note that where peer-to-peer training is adopted, peer trainers face several competing pressures, including high workloads and multiple responsibilities (Okyere et al., 2017). This is illustrated by the following quote from a CHW supervisor in Ghana who stated: 'The workload is too much for me here. I am the administrator, accountant, and consultant and I also train and supervise the other staff so you can imagine what I am going through. There is no motivation for doing all these tasks' (Okyere et al., 2017, p. 16).

Challenges Related to Trainers and Supervisors

A 2018 study found that high CHW satisfaction in Uganda was associated with frequent contact with supervisors, positive relationships, the opportunity for feedback, and the demonstration of mutual respect (Ludwick et al., 2018). However, supervision of health workers in LMICs has traditionally been carried out in a technocratic and controlling fashion, emphasizing the importance of inspection (Thakral, 2015). Genuine supervision, in which 'values, beliefs, motivations... and identities are emphasised' (Crow, 2012, p. 235) has been prohibited from occurring due to 'the entrenched authoritarian supervisory paradigm' (Nkomazana et al., 2016, p. 2, quoting Marquez & Keane, 2002). This has led to researchers such as Couper et al. (2018) to call for supervision for health workers in Africa to focus more on clinical mentorship than administration (Couper et al., 2018). However, this will require a paradigm shift in order to facilitate genuine supportive supervision in many LMICs (Clements et al., 2007).

A further key problem related to supervisors is that many lack formal training in good supervisory practices and techniques. Often CHW supervisors can be poorly organized and unaware of the needs of their supervisees (van Ginneken et al., 2010). One such example was highlighted in study by Crispin et al. (2012), which found that CHW supervisors often lack the skills required to carry out their role effectively. Similarly, a study by Ndima et al. (2015) found that several CHW supervisors in Mozambique had never received training in good supervisory practices. One was quoted as saying: 'I am supervisor since the APE (CHW) programme was revitalized here, but I have never been trained' (Ndima et al., 2015, p. 6). This study also found that CHWs felt their supervisors largely focused on fault-finding, which in turn was demotivating (Ndima et al., 2015).

These issues highlight the need to provide training on how to be a supervisor. This was found to be beneficial in a study by Nkomazana et al. (2016), who conducted co-operative inquiry groups with supervisors of a primary healthcare programme in rural Botswana. This investigation revealed that after a period of reflection, supervisors felt they needed to change their supervisory style to incorporate values such as transparency, encouragement, holistic support, collaboration and teamwork (Nkomazana et al., 2016). There is therefore a need to respond to the call by Winters et al. (2017), for greater interdisciplinary collaboration between the field of health sciences and education (Winters et al., 2017). Drawing upon the extensive research already conducted on good mentorship in the field of education could prove valuable in helping to guide the design and implementation of CHW supervisor training. As highlighted by Bush et al. (1996), qualities of a good mentor such as active listening, good interpersonal skills, commitment to their role and regular feedback were those most appreciated by mentees (Bush et al., 1996). Bush et al. also noted 'formal hierarchical relationships were alien to an effective mentoring relationship' (Bush et al., 1996, p. 132). Similarly, Crow suggests a socio-constructivist approach to mentorship in education, which places emphasis on learning in which 'inquiry, sense making and reflection are foundational' (Crow, 2012, p. 233). Importantly, Barnett and O'Mahony (2008) suggest that a good mentor should encourage reflection. This involves reflection on exemplary models of practice and reflection on their own practice (Barnett and O'Mahony, 2008). Such qualities and features should be emphasized, encouraged, and evaluated during supervisor training programmes.

Another problem relates to how CHW trainers and supervisors are selected. This is important, since it has been suggested that the professional background of supervisors might influence their supervisory style. For example, trainers in South Africa who previously worked in clerical roles took an administrative approach towards their role, whereas those with a background in counselling focused more on providing emotional support (Daniels et al., 2010). It is therefore important to consider the ability of the supervisor to relate to the needs of the CHW when undertaking supervisor selection (Duthie et al., 2012). The importance of this was demonstrated in a 2013 study by Kok and Muula, where CHWs in Malawi felt the supervision process was hindered by a lack of recognition and respect from supervisors (Kok & Muula, 2013). One of the CHWs interviewed as part of this study stated: 'We are voiceless in this health system' (Kok & Muula, 2013, p. 8).

Disjointed Training and Supervisory Frameworks

Where supervision programmes do exist they are commonly unstructured and lack a framework for delivery and evaluation. The patchwork landscape of CHW providers, ranging from NGOs to governments, compounds this issue and makes it challenging to navigate the field. Different providers have different ways of conducting supervisory practice, and are often not accountable to anyone.

Kok and Muula (2013) noted that there was no framework in place for giving feedback to CHWs in Malawi as part of a training and supervision programme for CHWs

(Kok & Muula, 2013). A lack of feedback from supervisors and low frequency of supervision was also associated with greater rates of attrition among volunteer CHWs in Kenya (Ngugi et al., 2018). Similarly, a study by De Neve et al. (2017) revealed that due to the disjointed provider networks in Swaziland, CHW programmes focusing on the delivery of supportive supervision for HIV care were piecemeal and often took vertical approaches to delivery (De Neve et al., 2017). Taking a more holistic approach to supervision and considering how it is embedded within the broader health system is therefore important.

Infrastructure Barriers

There are also logistical barriers that hinder supervision, such as poor transport access in rural areas during the rainy season (Kok & Muula, 2013). This can mean CHWs are unable to travel to 'in-person' supervisory sessions if roads become unfit for travel. Further, CHWs often have to travel long distances in order to receive supervision. One Tanzanian CHW in a study by Greenspan et al. (2013) highlighted the difficulties in distance by stating: 'I know they [health workers] have more expertise than me, but since we are located very far [from a health centre], for me it is very important to be supervised during the [service] delivery process' (Greenspan et al., 2013, p. 9).

Competing Interests

The ability of CHWs to attend supervision sessions could also be impacted by their busy personal and professional lives. For example, volunteer CHWs will have other competing interests to balance alongside their roles as health providers, such as their regular jobs. This was highlighted in a study by Greenspan et al. (2013), where CHWs struggled to fit supervision into their daily routine: 'As you know, this is a volunteer position. Therefore, we need time to do our personal work' (Greenspan et al., 2013, p. 10).

Funding

A 2017 study by Taylor et al. found that government funding for comprehensive CHW programmes is lacking across many LMICs, especially in sub-Saharan Africa. Given that the benefits of ongoing training and supervision are not always immediately apparent, other areas such as medicine procurement, or equipment supplies, are often prioritized by those managing CHW programmes for 'quick wins'.

In light of the numerous challenges outlined above, alternative strategies are required to help to support the delivery of supervision for CHWs. Given the high ownership of mobile phones in many LMIC settings (including Uganda, where mobile phone ownership stands at 55% of the total population) (World Bank, 2018), their use has been suggested as one way to address some of the challenges surrounding the provision of supervision for CHWs (O'Donovan et al., 2015). Their use could help to improve access, remove infrastructural barriers and help to improve the structure and educational quality of supervision, by drawing upon the inherent social networks of CHWs (DeRenzi et al., 2011; Labrique et al., 2013; Mwendwa, 2018).

Although the use of mobile technologies to facilitate the training and supervision of CHWs will be discussed in significant detail in other chapters, I will provide a brief overview in the next section of this chapter as to their potential benefits, challenges, and opportunities by drawing upon the existing literature.

The Use of Mobile Technologies to Assist CHW Supervision

mHealth can be broadly defined as 'mobile computing, medical sensor, and communications technologies for healthcare' (O'Donovan et al., 2015, p. 33). As outlined by Labrique et al., mobile technologies have several roles in assisting health system strengthening, one of which is to support the education and training of health professionals (Labrique et al., 2013).

To date much of the literature on the role of mobile technologies to assist in the training and education of CHWs has focused on a technocentric approach towards evaluation (Winters et al., 2017). As a result, the popularity of mobile phones as a supervisory adjunct is largely driven by the promise of improved data collection and the ability to deliver supervision at scale. While these benefits are undoubtedly promising, there is almost a complete absence of research regarding how the use of mobile technologies might benefit the most marginalized groups of CHWs and how they might facilitate learning.

In a systematic scoping review by Winters et al. (2018), the role of mobile technologies to facilitate education and training for CHWs was evaluated. Significantly, of the 24 studies where mobile technologies were used to support CHWs' training and education, only four referred to formal theories of learning from educational research. In this article, the authors suggest that much of the existing literature suffers from a 'reductionist view of learning that underestimates the complexities of the relationship between pedagogy and technology' (Winters et al., 2018, p. 1). Many of the studies included in the review used measures of information exposure as a proxy for learning. Winters et al. caution against these simplistic approaches towards training and education, since it is unclear as to how they might empower CHWs, or how they help us to understand how learning takes place. One such example of a simplistic mHealth supervisory intervention was a study in Zambia (Biemba et al., 2017). Here, CHWs used mobile phones to send weekly reports to their supervisors. In return they received SMS messages to invite them for mentorship sessions. In this example, mobile technologies have been used as an administrative tool, rather than a pedagogical function. Furthermore, although significant emphasis was placed on data collection and reporting, less emphasis was placed on capacity building and learning.

Specifically, one particular area of CHW education and training that could be supported by mobile technologies is supervision. For example, mobile technologies could be used to support reflective and interactive learning through real-time feedback by a remote supervisor, or peer-to-peer support via instant messaging services. Such uses of mobile technologies have been documented in the education literature more broadly. However, they have been under researched with regards to CHW supervision. In a systematic scoping review published in 2018, only seven studies that evaluated the use of mobile technologies to facilitate CHW supervision in LMIC settings were identified (O'Donovan et al., 2018). Of these, three used simplistic one-way SMS messages, with only one study by Henry et al. (2016) focusing on how mobile technologies might facilitate a more dialogical form of learning, through peer-to-peer interaction via WhatsApp in Kenya (Henry et al., 2016). There was a lack of a description across all studies with regards to how supervision was defined by the authors or how they positioned their work with regards to the existing literature on m-learning. This has led to calls for greater collaboration between members of the health and education research communities.

It is also important to note that the use of mobile assisted approaches is not without their challenges. In a study by Mwendwa (2016), it was found that although an SMS supervisory system helped programme managers keep track of CHWs activities and allowed for data to be quickly sent to the MoH, CHWs expressed several areas of dissatisfaction (Mwendwa, 2016). For example, in one focus discussion group, CHWs stated: 'We need to have more supervision when using RapidSMS. We have not used this technology before so it takes long to learn how to send the messages' (Mwendwa, 2016, p. 44).

Other issues included dissatisfaction with the automated messaging service, difficulties in contacting supervisors and feedback being in English rather than the local language. For example, one CHW expressed their frustration with the automated messaging service, since they felt it did not adequately answer areas of concern or fully address their needs as learners: 'The system should point out where we make mistakes; I am tired of sending messages without success' (Mwendwa, 2016, p. 46).

Similarly, several challenges were highlighted regarding an mHealth project in Nepal with rural CHWs. The authors of this study highlighted the importance of ensuring the suitability of technology to the local context, and bringing together key stakeholders to decide on the goals of the programme prior to commencement. Indeed previous research has noted that many mobile-assisted education and training programmes for CHWs fail to consider the contextual and cultural factors which are crucial to their overall acceptance and long-term use. Tariq and Durrani (2018) suggest the need for a paradigm shift away from the 'techno-deterministic design focus' on mobile-based interventions, towards one informed by context.

Finally, it is important to note that the challenges of a mobile-assisted approach are not restricted to individuals. In 2011, the government of Uganda issued a moratorium on all mHealth projects within the country due to a concern with the large number of pilot projects that failed to scale and integrate with government systems. It is therefore important that those responsible for establishing mHealth-based interventions work with key stakeholders at every level, from the community through to government policy makers, to help maximize chances of adoption.

Conclusion

This chapter provides a historical background to CHW programmes, as well as outlining how training and supervision for healthcare professionals more broadly has evolved over time. These topics are important to understand since they have ultimately helped to shape the current field of CHW training and supervision. I then outlined some of the key challenges facing modern CHW programmes, specifically with regards to training and supervision. Finally, I concluded by highlighting some of the key opportunities that could play a role in helping to address some of these challenges, such as the role of mobile technologies. Through this process I have begun to lay the foundations to help you understand the complexities of this fragmented, contested, and important field of study and practice.

To date, CHW programmes have largely followed a training and supervision model based around 'information dissemination', which largely prioritizes knowledge and skills acquisition. Whilst knowledgeable and skilled CHWs are undoubtedly important for the safety and well-being of the individuals they serve, there remains a relative paucity of research on how local knowledge can be incorporated into training and supervision programmes. By using more participatory approaches in the design of CHW training and supervision, programmes are more likely to be responsive to the needs of CHWs, and the communities they serve.

Finally, it is important to note that whatever approach to training and supervision is adopted, CHWs must remain at the heart of all programmes.

References

Ballard, M., Schwarz, R., Johnson, A., Church, S., Palazuelos, D., McCormick, L., et al. (2018). *Practitioner Expertise to Optimize Community Health Systems: Harnessing Operational Insight*. CHW Central, New York.

Barnett, B.G. & O'Mahony, G.R. (2008). Mentoring and coaching programs for the professional development of school leaders. In: J. Lumby, G. Crow, & P. Pashiardis (Eds). *International Handbook on the Preparation and Development of School Leaders*. New York, Routledge, pp. 232–262.

Bernard, J.M. & Goodyear, R.K. (1992). *Fundamentals of Clinical Supervision*. Boston, Allyn & Bacon.

Biemba, G., Chiluba, B., Yeboah-Antwi, K., Silavwe, V., Lunze, K., Mwale, R.K., et al. (2017). A mobile-based community health management information system for community health workers and their supervisors in 2 districts of Zambia. *Global Health: Science and Practice*, 5, 486–494.

Bosch-Capblanch, X. & Marceau, C. (2014). Training, supervision and quality of care in selected integrated community case management (iCCM) programmes: A scoping review of programmatic evidence. *Journal of Global Health*, 4, 020403–020403.

Bush, T., Coleman, M., Wall, D., & West-Burnham, J. (1996). Mentoring and continuing professional development. In: H. Hagger & D. MacIntyre (Eds). *Mentors in Schools*. London, Routledge, pp. 120–143.

Clements, C.J., Streefland, P.H., & Malau, C. (2007). Supervision in primary health care—can it be carried out effectively in developing countries? *Current Drug Safety*, 2, 19–23.

Cometto, G., Ford, N., Pfaffman-Zambruni, J., Akl, E.A., Lehmann, U., Mcpake, B., et al. (2018). Health policy and system support to optimise community health worker programmes: An abridged WHO guideline. *Lancet Global Health*, 6, e1397–e1404.

Couper, I., Ray, S., Blaauw, D., Ng'wena, G., Muchiri, L., Oyungu, E., et al. (2018). Curriculum and training needs of mid-level health workers in Africa: A situational review from Kenya, Nigeria, South Africa and Uganda. *BMC Health Services Research*, 18, 553.

Crigler, L., Gergen, J., & Perry, H. (2013). *Supervision of Community Health Workers*. Available from: https://www.mchip.net/sites/default/files/mchipfiles/09_CHW_Supervision.pdf

Crispin, N., Wamae, A., Ndirangu, M., Wamalwa, D., Wangalwa, G., Watako, P., et al. (2012). Effects of selected socio-demographic characteristics of community health workers on performance of home visits during pregnancy: A cross-sectional study in Busia District, Kenya. *Global Journal of Health Science*, 4, 78.

Crow, G.M. (2012). A critical-constructivist perspective on mentoring. In: S. Fletcher & C.A. Mullen (Eds). *SAGE Handbook of Mentoring and Coaching in Education*. London, Sage.

Daniels, K., Nor, B., Jackson, D., Ekström, E.-C., & Doherty, T. (2010). Supervision of community peer counsellors for infant feeding in South Africa: An exploratory qualitative study. *Human Resources for Health*, 8, 6.

De Neve, J.-W., Garrison-Desany, H., Andrews, K.G., Sharara, N., Boudreaux, C., Gill, R., et al. (2017). Harmonization of community health worker programs for HIV: A four-country qualitative study in Southern Africa. *PLoS Medicine*, 14.

Derenzi, B., Borriello, G., Jackson, J., Kumar, V.S., Parikh, T. S., Virk, P., et al. (2011). Mobile phone tools for field-based health care workers in low-income countries. *Mount Sinai Journal of Medicine: A Journal of Translational and Personalized Medicine*, 78, 406–418.

Duthie, P., Hahn, J., Philippi, E., & Sanchez, C. (2012). Keys to successful community health worker supervision. *American Journal of Health Education*, 43, 62–64.

George, A.S., Lefevre, A.E., Schleiff, M., Mancuso, A., Sacks, E., & Sarriot, E. (2018). Hubris, humility and humanity: Expanding evidence approaches for improving and sustaining community health programmes. *BMJ Global Health*, 3, e000811.

Greenspan, J.A., Mcmahon, S.A., Chebet, J.J., Mpunga, M., Urassa, D.P., & Winch, P.J. (2013). Sources of community health worker motivation: A qualitative study in Morogoro Region, Tanzania. *Human Resources for Health*, 11(52), 1–14.

Henry, J.V., Winters, N., Lakati, A., Oliver, M., Geniets, A., Mbae, S.M., et al. (2016). Enhancing the supervision of community health workers with WhatsApp mobile messaging: Qualitative findings from 2 low-resource settings in Kenya. *Global Health: Science and Practice*, e-ghsp-d-15-00386.

Hernández, A.R., Hurtig, A.-K., Dahlblom, K., & San Sebastián, M. (2014). More than a checklist: A realist evaluation of supervision of mid-level health workers in rural Guatemala. *BMC Health Services Research*, 14, 112.

Hill, Z., Dumbaugh, M., Benton, L., Källander, K., Strachan, D., Ten Asbroek, A., et al. (2014). Supervising community health workers in low-income countries—a review of impact and implementation issues. *Global Health Action*, 7, 24085.

Kadushin, A. & Harkness, D. (2014). *Supervision in Social Work* (Fifth Edition). New York, Columbia University Press.

Kilminster, S., Cottrell, D., Grant, J., & Jolly, B. (2007). AMEE Guide No. 27: Effective educational and clinical supervision. *Medical Teacher*, 29, 2–19.

Kok, M.C. & Muula, A.S. (2013). Motivation and job satisfaction of health surveillance assistants in Mwanza, Malawi: An explorative study. *Malawi Medical Journal*, 25, 5–11.

Labrique, A.B., Vasudevan, L., Kochi, E., Fabricant, R., & Mehl, G. (2013). mHealth innovations as health system strengthening tools: 12 common applications and a visual framework. *Global Health: Science and Practice*, 1, 160–171.

Leslie, H.H., Gage, A., Nsona, H., Hirschhorn, L.R., & Kruk, M.E. (2016). Training and supervision did not meaningfully improve quality of care for pregnant women or sick children in sub-Saharan Africa. *Health Affairs*, 35, 1716–1724.

Limb, M. (2016). World will lack 18 million health workers by 2030 without adequate investment, warns UN. *British Medical Journal*, 354, i5169.

Ludwick, T., Turyakira, E., Kyomuhangi, T., Manalili, K., Robinson, S., & Brenner, J.L. (2018). Supportive supervision and constructive relationships with healthcare workers support CHW performance: Use of a qualitative framework to evaluate CHW programming in Uganda. *Human Resources for Health*, 16, 11.

Marquez, L. & Keane, L. (2002). *Making supervision supportive and sustainable: New approaches to old problems. Supplement to Population Reports.* Washington D.C., Maximizing Access and Quality (MAQ) Initiative.

Mwendwa, P. (2016). Assessing the fit of RapidSMS for maternal and new-born health: Perspectives of community health workers in rural Rwanda. *Development in Practice*, 26, 38–51.

Mwendwa, P. (2018). What encourages community health workers to use mobile technologies for health interventions? Emerging lessons from rural Rwanda. *Development Policy Review*, 36, 111–129.

Ndima, S.D., Sidat, M., Ormel, H., Kok, M.C., & Taegtmeyer, M. (2015). Supervision of community health workers in Mozambique: A qualitative study of factors influencing motivation and programme implementation. *Human Resources for Health*, 13, 63.

Ngugi, A.K., Nyaga, L.W., Lakhani, A., Agoi, F., Hanselman, M., Lugogo, G., et al. (2018). Prevalence, incidence and predictors of volunteer community health worker attrition in Kwale County, Kenya. *BMJ Global Health*, 3, e000750.

Nkomazana, O., Mash, R., Wojczewski, S., Kutalek, R., & Phaladze, N. (2016). How to create more supportive supervision for primary healthcare: Lessons from Ngamiland district of Botswana: Co-operative inquiry group. *Global Health Action*, 9, 31263.

O'Donovan, J., Bersin, A., & O'Donovan, C. (2015). The effectiveness of mobile health (mHealth) technologies to train healthcare professionals in developing countries: a review of the literature. *BMJ Innovations*, 1, 33–36.

O'Donovan, J., O'Donovan, C., Kuhn, I., Sachs, S.E., & Winters, N. (2018). Ongoing training of community health workers in low-income and middle-income countries: A systematic scoping review of the literature. *BMJ Open*, 8, e021467.

Okyere, E., Mwanri, L., & Ward, P. (2017). Is task-shifting a solution to the health workers' shortage in Northern Ghana? *PloS ONE*, 12(3), e0174631.

One Million CHWs (2014). *'What Do We Really Know?'—An Integrated Analysis of Current Research on Community Health Worker Training.* Available from: http://1millionhealthworkers.

org/files/2014/07/mPowering_IntegratedCurricAnalysis_1mCHW_Formatted-2.compressed.pdf

Palazuelos, D., Farmer, P.E., & Mukherjee, J. (2018). Community health and equity of outcomes: The Partners in Health experience. *Lancet Global Health*, 6, e491–e493.

Pfeiffer, J. & Chapman, R.R. (2019). NGOs, austerity, and universal health coverage in Mozambique. *Globalization and Health*, 15, 1–6.

Roberton, T., Applegate, J., Lefevre, A.E., Mosha, I., Cooper, C.M., Silverman, M., et al. (2015). Initial experiences and innovations in supervising community health workers for maternal, newborn, and child health in Morogoro region, Tanzania. *Human Resources for Health*, 13, 19.

Rosales, M., Hedrick, J., Cherian, D., Amet, K.K., Walumbe, E., Dunbar, G., et al. (2015). *Supervising Illiterate Community Health Workers in South Sudan to Deliver Integrated Community Case Management Services for Newborns and Children*. Available from: https://www.worldvision.org/wp-content/uploads/2017/03/OR-Final-Sudan-Sudan-report-02_19-_2015.pdf

Schneider, H. (2019). *Assessing Community Health Worker Programme Governance: A Guiding Framework*. CHW Central. Available from: https://www.chwcentral.org/blog/assessing-community-health-worker-programme-governance-guiding-framework

Simon, S., Chu, K., Frieden, M., Candrinho, B., Ford, N., Schneider, H., et al. (2009). An integrated approach of community health worker support for HIV/AIDS and TB care in Angonia district, Mozambique. *BMC International Health and Human Rights*, 9, 13.

Tariq, A. & Durrani, S. (2018). One size does not fit all: The importance of contextually sensitive mHealth strategies for frontline female health workers. In: E. Baulch, J. Watkins, & A. Tariq (Eds). *mHealth Innovation in Asia: Grassroots Challenges and Practical Interventions*. Dordrecht, Springer.

Tavrow, P., Kim, Y.-M., & Malianga, L. (2002). Measuring the quality of supervisor–provider interactions in health care facilities in Zimbabwe. *International Journal for Quality in Health Care*, 14, 57–66.

Thakral, S. (2015). The historical context of modern concept of supervision. *Journal of Emerging Trends in Educational Research and Policy Studies*, 6(1), 79–88.

The World Bank (2018). *Mobile cellular subscriptions (per 100 people)*. Available from: https://data.worldbank.org/indicator/IT.CEL.SETS.P2

The World Health Organization (2008). *Training for Mid-level Managers (MLM)—Supportive Supervision*. Available from: http://www.who.int/immunization/documents/MLM_module4.pdf

Tomlinson, J. (2015). Using clinical supervision to improve the quality and safety of patient care: A response to Berwick and Francis. *BMC Medical Education*, 15, 103.

Van Ginneken, N., Lewin, S., & Berridge, V. (2010). The emergence of community health worker programmes in the late apartheid era in South Africa: An historical analysis. *Social Science & Medicine*, 71, 1110–1118.

Winters, N., Oliver, M., & Langer, L. (2017). Can mobile health training meet the challenge of 'measuring better'? *Comparative Education*, 53, 115–131.

Winters, N., Langer, L., & Geniets, A. (2018). Scoping review assessing the evidence used to support the adoption of mobile health (mHealth) technologies for the education and training of community health workers (CHWs) in low-income and middle-income countries. *BMJ Open*, 8, e019827.

5

Digital Health Interventions for Community Health Worker Training, Ongoing Education, and Supportive Supervision

Insights from a Human-Centred Design Approach

Beatrice Wasunna and Isaac Holeman

Introduction

Despite proclamations that mobile technologies have the potential to transform health service delivery (Mahmud et al., 2010; Kay, Santos, & Takane, 2011; Labrique et al., 2013; Agarwal et al., 2015; Ilozumba et al., 2018) and studies that have demonstrated ways in which mobile infrastructure can be used to improve health outcomes in low resource settings (Lester et al., 2010; Pop-Eleches et al., 2011; Chib et al., 2015; Feldacker et al., 2019), it has often proved difficult to establish programmes that can be reproduced or conducted at scale. The difficulties experienced in mHealth projects are often attributed to simplistic assumptions about local contextual factors, rapid technological and political change, or because scaling up from small-scale trials presents too many complexities (see Holeman & Kane, 2019). As discussed in the chapter by Panjabi et al. (Chapter 2), the potential role of technology in community health worker (CHW) education and training must be delicately balanced between the rhetoric of what's possible and the realities on the ground in hard-to-reach communities.

There has been a call for a more flexible, contextually driven process for designing such complex technological systems. Human-centred design (HCD) represents a flexible, yet disciplined and repeatable approach to innovation that puts people at the centre of the design activity. It prioritizes human aspirations and ordinary experiences when imagining and implementing complex systems, services, or products. Human-centred design has become central to how Medic, the non-profit organization where we work, approaches innovation for global health.

This chapter focuses on Medic's approach to designing and deploying digital health tools for ongoing training and supervision of CHWs in the delivery of door-step care.

Beatrice Wasunna and Isaac Holeman, *Digital Health Interventions for Community Health Worker Training, Ongoing Education, and Supportive Supervision* In: *Training for Community Health*. Edited by: Anne Geniets, James O'Donovan, Laura Hakimi, and Niall Winters, Oxford University Press. © Oxford University Press 2021. DOI: 10.1093/oso/9780198866244.003.0005

The first part of the chapter introduces Medic's Community Health Toolkit and describes the specific way in which HCD has been applied to mobile health. The second section of this chapter focuses on CHW training and the considerations for training on digital health tools. Drawing on action design approach, and iterative, reflective methodology that also prioritizes local experience, the chapter then provides an example of training CHWs in Nepal, commonly referred to as 'female community health volunteers' (FCHVs), on Medic digital heath tools. The example sets out a description of the digital health tools as well as user insights on acceptability and usability of these tools. The chapter proceeds with a brief discussion on the role of supervision in CHW performance management and opportunities to leverage digital health tools to strengthen supportive supervision.

Medic's Organizational Context

In low-resource settings, CHWs are front-line providers who shoulder the health service delivery burden. Increasingly, mobile technologies are developed, tested, and deployed with CHWs to facilitate tasks and improve outcomes. Medic is a non-profit organization that uses communication technologies to improve the health of underserved and disconnected communities. We build mobile and web tools for health workers (Figure 5.1), helping them provide better care that reaches everyone. All of Medic's code and resources are collaboratively developed and released as public goods as part of the Community Health Toolkit (CHT) open-source project (https://communityhealthtoolkit.org/). The CHT provides resources to design, build, and deploy the digital tools CHWs need to reach the poorest and most marginalized. By rethinking who health workers are, where care is delivered, and what makes up a healthcare system, it supports a new model of care that brings health services to everyone and has been known to significantly improve health outcomes. The technologies and resources in the CHT have been co-designed with local health teams to support a remote workforce.

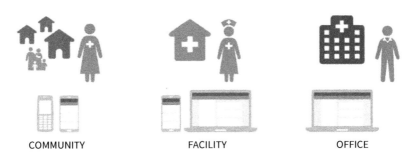

COMMUNITY   FACILITY   OFFICE

Figure 5.1 Medic tools.
Adapted with permission from Medic's Community Health Toolkit. Copyright © Medic 2020.

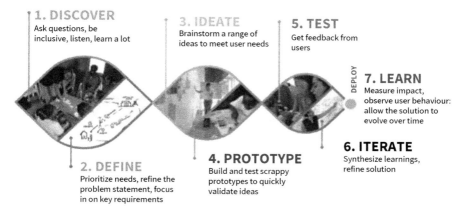

1. DISCOVER
Ask questions, be inclusive, listen, learn a lot

3. IDEATE
Brainstorm a range of ideas to meet user needs

5. TEST
Get feedback from users

DEPLOY

7. LEARN
Measure impact, observe user behaviour: allow the solution to evolve over time

6. ITERATE
Synthesize learnings, refine solution

2. DEFINE
Prioritize needs, refine the problem statement, focus in on key requirements

4. PROTOTYPE
Build and test scrappy prototypes to quickly validate ideas

Figure 5.2 Seven steps of the human-centred design approach at Medic.
Adapted with permission from Medic's design SoPs. Copyright © Medic 2020.

The CHT is a free open-source toolkit to advance universal health coverage through shared technologies and resources. The Application Framework helps people delivering care in hard-to-reach areas. It supports CHWs, nurses, and managers. The CHT currently supports 25,000 health workers serving 14 million people.

Medic's approach to mobile technology for health (mHealth) prioritizes the end users of its tools, through the human centred design approach. The practice of HCD begins with cultivating empathy for our users and understanding their needs, motivations, strengths, and priorities (Figure 5.2). These insights ensure appealing tools for community health volunteers, nurses, patients, and Ministry of Health. They further facilitate designing of workflows that integrate daily practices in the community towards attaining highest health impact. The goal of this process is to develop an interface and workflow for CHW interactive SMS messaging with clients, app functionality to support and guide CHW responses to SMS, and an interface and workflow for supervisor monitoring and quality assurance of CHW-client SMS. This HCD approach features shadowing of home visits, user testing of mock-up versions of the application, and consultations with government staff overseeing CHW service delivery.

Human Centred-Design for Iteration Planning

HCD is an approach to innovation that puts people at the centre of activity, and uses a range of methods from the social sciences to rapidly generate evidence about the human dimensions of design projects, enabling a more evidence-based, iterative process.

According to the International Standards Organization (ISO, 2010), HCD is a complex practice characterized by: user involvement throughout design and development; user-centred evaluation; an interactive process; attention to the whole user experience, including the context in which the user finds his/herself; and multidisciplinary skills and perspectives. At its heart, HCD privileges stakeholder participation, augmenting human skills, and an explicit understanding of users, tasks, and environment.

Medic's well documented HCD practice (see Holeman & Kane, 2019) incorporates three key activities: (1) an initial design visit to define contextual requirements and determine a suitable workflow; (2) system usage analysis and adaptation; and (3) user feedback sessions undertaken following deployment. The data collected in activities 1 and 3 are primarily qualitative, whereas data on system usage is primarily quantitative as described in the user feedback section of this chapter.

Training of CHWs

Training is a key component of CHW programmes. There are varying approaches adopted to training CHWs across community health programmes (O'Donovan et al., 2018). These range from short-term training to more long-term certificate programmes. Training content also varies significantly based on the educational qualifications of CHWs and the required competencies for their roles and responsibilities, ranging from use of nationally produced training modules to locally tailored curricula, residential courses, or mobile training teams. Despite the adoption of digital health interventions for community health programmes, there remains little evidence of training CHWs on these tools (Winters et al., 2019). At Medic, training of CHWs within mHealth projects is undertaken in collaboration with implementing partners. Prior to the training sessions information is obtained on CHW characteristics to understand the demographic dynamics of the group. This chapter describes the deployment of Medic's CHT in Nepal.

Considerations for Training CHWs on Digital Health Tools

Several demographic, personal characteristics, and work context factors should be considered when training CHWs on digital health tools.

The majority of CHW programmes consist of both middle-aged and elderly community members. A good majority are retired professionals and elderly persons that may require patience and empathy from the trainers to ensure that they grasp key components of digital health tools. Furthermore these CHWs may require additional time during the training to ascertain that the key objectives of the training have been achieved across all groups. Studies have emphasized the importance of age, level of education, and previous technology use as factors to consider when designing digital health training programmes targeted at CHWs (Jimoh et al., 2012; Jennings et al., 2013).

The CHW level of education varies within community health programmes. Some of the individuals nominated as CHWs by the communities may not have the minimum numeracy and literacy to complete documentation or understanding of key concepts required during training. Additionally, the language of instruction during the training is key in addressing some of the issues around understanding of training content. Local language/vernacular may be preferable for training CHWs in some settings to overcome some of the limitations arising from low literacy levels. Furthermore, it is important to work with local communities to identify culturally appropriate teaching techniques as well as tools and skills appropriate for low-literacy communities with limited resources and technology.

During training, there are likely to be variations in years of experience among CHWs. Trainers should anticipate that the CHWs with several years of experience are likely to be more familiar with the content of the forms and are likely to progress quickly though the workflows, unlike those who are new to the CHW programme. Trainers should take into consideration the variations in CHW experience to accommodate these variations in experience.

An assumption of digital health interventions is that with the proliferation of mobile phones this translates into improved phone coverage in low and middle-income countries (LMICs) where CHW programmes are deployed. However, it is not uncommon to find CHWs with limited or no exposure to the use of mobile phones, whether basic feature or smart/android phones. Therefore prior to training on digital health tools, trainers and implementing teams should assess the exposure and provide CHWs with an opportunity to explore the mobile devices prior to the training activities.

Sensitization of CHWs prior to the introduction of digital health solutions is important for uptake and sustainability. Specifically, prior to training it can be useful in demystifying some of the misconceptions around transitioning to digital health tools from paper-based tools. CHWs may perceive digital tools as additional work or as a disruption to their daily routine.

As mentioned earlier, CHW age is a key consideration for training on digital health tools. Trainers should integrate the principles of adult learning when training CHWs on digital health tools. These include: (1) a need to know why they are learning; (2) motivation to learn by the need to solve problems; (3) respect and building upon previous experience; (4) adopting learning approaches that match CHW background and diversity; and (5) active participation in the learning process.

From the above considerations on training CHWs on digital health tools, trainers and implementers should be guided by Paulo Freire's (2000) principle of recognizing that training and education can and ought to be fundamentally about empowerment of CHWs. By equipping CHWs with digital health tools, training not only provides them with the knowledge on specific health areas but also conveys respect and recognition from the communities they serve.

Training of CHWs on Digital Health Tools to Improve Maternal, Neonatal and Child Health (MNCH) in Nepal

Background on Nepal's Health System (MNCH Statistics) and Context on the National FCHV Network

Contextual factors play a critical role in the design of effective CHW training programmes on digital health interventions. An understanding of the contextual factors in which CHW interventions operate is an important prerequisite for the design of successful digital health interventions (Haines et al., 2007; Standing et al., 2008; Palazuelos et al., 2013). Nepal has made significant progress in reducing maternal and child mortality since it began providing community-based service delivery 30 years ago. Despite a decade-long, armed conflict, political instability, and the country's vulnerability to natural disaster, Nepal achieved MDG goal 4 along with a sharp reduction in poverty (Sudyumna & Kitzmuller, 2017), and these successes are often lauded internationally. Political will, coordinated efforts by the government, and increased financial investment by international partners may have contributed to the improvement, but community based programmes led by a huge national volunteer workforce known as Female Community Health Volunteers (FCHVs) also played a vital role.

In 2016, 40% of births were delivered at home (NDHS, 2016). Gaps in coverage for essential health interventions are most significant in mountainous areas, for people who have the least formal education, and for poorer families.

The Nepal Demographic and Health Survey (NDHS) reported 84% of women who gave birth in the five years before the survey received antenatal care (ANC) from a skilled provider, a 25-percentage point increase from 2011 (NDHS, 2016). Sixty-nine per cent of women had at least four ANC visits (Figure 5.3).

The neonatal mortality rate was reported as 21 deaths per 1000 live births, while the under-five mortality rate is 39 deaths per 1000 live births. This means that 54% of all under-five deaths occur in the first month of life. Between 1996 and 2016, neonatal mortality fell from 50 to 21 deaths per 1000 live births, infant mortality declined from 78 to 32 deaths per 1000 live births, and under-five mortality fell from 118 to 39 deaths per 1000 live births (Figure 5.4).

Recognizing these challenges, the Ministry of Health and Population (MoHP) in Nepal aims to improve access to care and outcomes for all citizens. Community health services are provided by the three cadres of community-level service providers (CLSPs): FCHVs, auxiliary nurse midwives (ANMs), and auxiliary health workers (AHWs). In 1988, the FCHV programme was initiated. Nepal has relied largely on this network of lay volunteers to act as connecters between the community and the healthcare system. During the last three decades, the role of the FCHVs has evolved and they have taken on various activities including health promotion, distribution of preventive health commodities, home-based healthcare provision, and support in national programmes such as vitamin A supplementation programme.

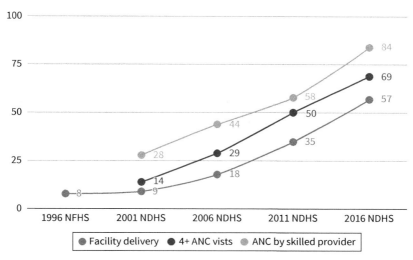

Figure 5.3 The percentage of women aged 15–49 years between 1996 and 2016.
Source: Data from Nepal Demographic and Health Survey, 2016.

Encompassing the lessons from past community level interventions, the role of FCHVs has now narrowed down to providing community based health promotion, early detection, education and counselling, distribution of preventive health commodities such as oral rehydration solution, zinc tablets, and supporting the MoHP in National vitamin A campaigns, immunization programmes, etc. Currently a network of over 50,000 FCHVs forms the backbone of Nepal's community health system, and Medic has been empowering this health workforce with digital care coordination tools since 2012.

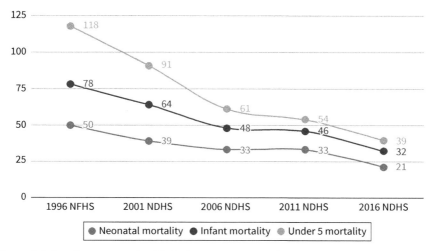

Figure 5.4 Deaths per 1000 live births between 1996 and 2016.
Source: Data from Nepal Demographic and Health Survey, 2016.

Adoption Model of the Nepalese Government

In Nepal, Medic has worked to harness technology for community healthcare co-ordination, health system strengthening, and FCHV empowerment since 2012. Building on efforts that began as a pilot in Baglung district in 2012 alongside a non-governmental organization (NGO) partner, One Heart Worldwide, the digital health programme has since been tested, refined, and scaled to over 12 districts. The iterations included both technical (minor changes to workflow) and programmatic improvements in the deployment approach.

In 2017, Medic and MoHP Nepal entered into a strategic partnership where the government funds and supports the implementation of the open-source tools, with capacity building (training of trainers) and technical support provided by Medic. This partnership allows sustainable scaling of the impact nationally, while ensuring government uptake and ownership at various levels. As Nepal restructures its government to a federal system and devolves greater authority to local levels of government, partnerships can be built directly with municipalities for the implementation and support of the mHealth programme at scale, and creative cost-sharing agreements can be adopted with them to ensure sustainability and programme continuity. In the future, it is envisioned that government staff will deploy and manage these systems.

Medic also provides broader systems strengthening and advocacy support to the government in various capacities. Medic currently serves as a member of the former National eHealth Technical Working Group, which was entrusted with operationalizing the National eHealth Strategy, including providing guidance to establish the framework for an integrated approach to information management in the health sector. Along with a range of community health stakeholders and partners, Medic is also currently supporting efforts to redefine the country's community health strategy. In service of interoperability, integrations of the toolkit with DHIS2, the Government of Nepal's central information management system are being explored.

The Community Health Toolkit in Nepal

The Community Health Toolkit is highly configurable; it enables decision support for front-line care, prioritization for home visits and follow-ups, smart messaging, and actionable analytics for managers (Figure 5.5). The tools built are free, open-source, and deployed at scale in the underserved communities in the last mile of healthcare.

A key component of the HCD approach during the initial exploratory phase is to undertake a situational analysis that includes an assessment of the ecosystem to identify infrastructural needs and identify optimal solutions for targeted users. In order to overcome connectivity and resource issues, the tools for familiar, basic phones work in communities with intermittent connectivity, leverage the most ubiquitous mobile infrastructure, and harness SMS as a communication and data channel. Medic

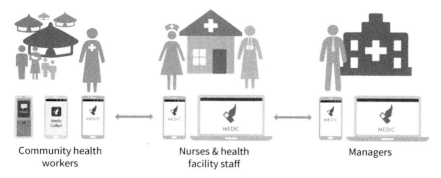

Community health   Nurses & health   Managers
workers   facility staff

Figure 5.5 Medic tools used by health workers in Nepal.
Reproduced with permission from Medic's Community Health Toolkit. Copyright © Medic 2020.

pioneered the use of parallel SIM card applications for healthcare in 2011, enabling
any basic phone to run applications for health workers.

In Nepal, FCHVs use Medic for SMS, or structured text messages on basic or
smartphones (Figure 5.6). This tool enables FCHVs to remotely register patients
for essential services, communicate vital events, receive antenatal and postnatal

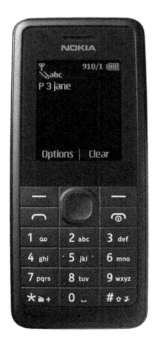
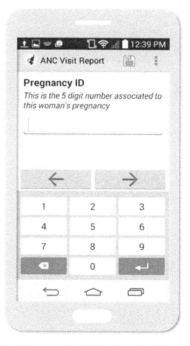

Figure 5.6 Medic for SMS (left-hand side); Medic collect for android (right-hand side).
Reproduced with permission from Medic's Community Health Toolkit. Copyright © Medic Mobile 2020.

care reminders, ensure safe deliveries, receive immunization reminders, track maternal and perinatal deaths, and improve health for mothers and newborns.

Facility staff utilize Medic Collect, an Android app that extends Open Data Kit (ODK) and includes forms with skip logic, location data, in-app data validation, and multimedia support. The facility-based health workers can submit data on Medic Collect by mobile Internet, Wi-Fi, or SMS as a backup. Health programme coordinators at municipalities, health officers at districts, and other management staff use the CHT web app, hosted either locally or in the cloud on desktops, laptops, tablets, or smartphones to view patient history and FCHV activity in real time. They also use powerful performance management dashboards that visualize activity and impact indicators, identify facilities and specific health workers who need more support, and help managers make programmatic decisions and resource allocations (Figures 5.7 and 5.8). All of these tools integrate seamlessly in real-time, connecting last-mile communities, FCHVs, and facilities.

Training FCHVs on Digital Health Tools

Medic adopts the Training of Trainers Model and strategy to engage health workers, municipal health coordinators, and health workers/district health officers/focal persons in the day-to-day monitoring of progress. While the orientation introduces them to the digital health programme, the specific mHealth tools, and other programmatic

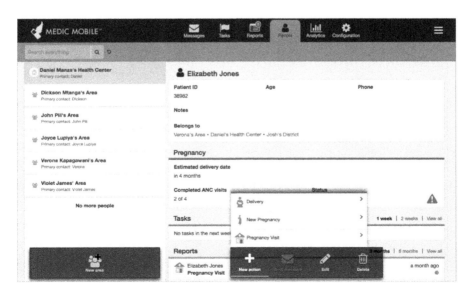

Figure 5.7 Medic Web App.
Reproduced with permission from Medic's Community Health Toolkit. Copyright © Medic 2020.

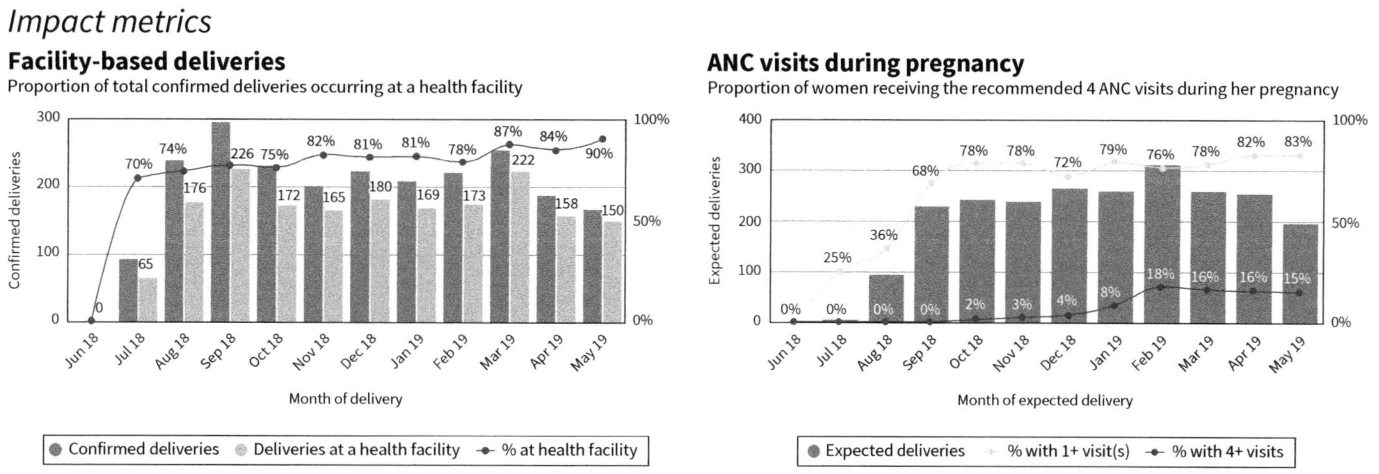

Impact metrics

Facility-based deliveries

Proportion of total confirmed deliveries occurring at a health facility

ANC visits during pregnancy

Proportion of women receiving the recommended 4 ANC visits during her pregnancy

Figure 5.8 Dashboard metric for ANC and facility based delivery.

Reproduced with permission from Medic's Community Health Toolkit. Copyright © Medic 2020.

elements, the training and capacity building focuses on mHealth programme-specific training, including how to use the mHealth tool for different health actions and for broader programme management and supervision. It also seeks to strengthen their ability to in turn train FCHVs and others on the tool going forward.

Deployment of Digital Tools to Improve Maternal and Child Health

Medic deployments in Nepal are supported by a team of 19 full-time staff in partnerships, project management, technical support, and design roles, and additional deployment support staff in the districts of implementation. Medic currently supports close to 8000 FCHVs with maternal and newborn care coordination tools through full coverage in 11 districts and several smaller scale deployments in three additional districts. Districts where Medic tools are currently deployed include: Baglung, Gorkha, Dhading, Ilam, Banke, Baitadi, Kanchanpur, Pyuthan, Bajura, Sindhupalchowk, Rasuwa, Sindhuli, and Sunsari (Figure 5.9).

   As implementation expands, it will also focus more deeply on the quality of deployments with a view to strengthening user engagement and providing an improved training experience to health facility users and FCHVs. Post-training, in addition to providing regular technical support to implementing partners, the field-based staff always try to ensure that grievances are dealt with effectively and in a timely way.

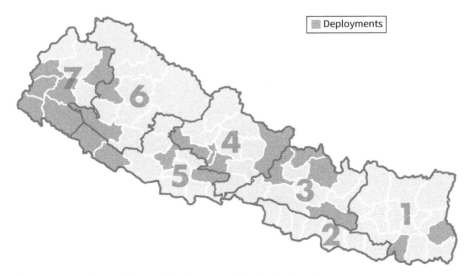

Figure 5.9 Medic training and deployment districts in Nepal.
Reproduced with permission from Medic's Community Health Toolkit. Copyright © Medic 2020.

Post-deployment activities also include:

- Training evaluations: there is a robust and well-defined evaluation process to monitor the effectiveness of each training delivered by Medic. It seeks to test, implement, and continually iterate on this in the future.
- Post-training follow up: there is conduct focused follow-up after training exercise in districts where the tool has been deployed. Qualitative and quantitative tools are used to better understand FCHV retention, experiences and challenges in using the toolkit. Findings from this light-touch, field follow-up often help to further refine deployments.
- Programme monitoring resources: access to the powerful analytics dashboard is provided to the authorities in the municipalities and health facilities. These tools help the decision makers and programme planners to provide feedback to the health cadres based on the live information displayed in the dashboard.
- Refresher training: Where appropriate, a structured refresher training curriculum and plan for our partners to implement is provided, so that they are able to effectively conduct these training at regular intervals, and increase and improve the quality of user engagement.
- Joint review meeting: there is regular participation in national, subnational, and local level joint review meetings. These forums provide an opportunity to share experience and guide the government team to better manage and use the tool.

User Feedback

Medic adopted an action design research (ADR) (Sein et al., 2011) approach in iteration planning. The ADR method complements a human-centred approach to the design, building, and deployment of projects, followed by a period of reflection and learning. Evaluation methods include both quantitative (system analyses) and qualitative (user feedback) assessments to identify potential iterations and the pathway to scale. Following deployment of the digital health tools (Figure 5.10), feedback sessions were undertaken with users to gain insights on the acceptability and usability, and to identify potential technological and deployment challenges.

Data collected from qualitative interviews are transcribed verbatim into Microsoft Word. Following the preliminary descriptive analysis, patterns were investigated, as well as linkages among views, experiences, and behaviours of the participants. There will be exploration of interpretations that might explain the observed patterns. Internal validity is ensured by audio-recording, verbatim transcription, and checking at random for accuracy and completeness of focus group discussions and in-depth interviews, and the qualitative data was analysed by two independent raters in order to increase reliability.

Following successful deployment, a user assessment of the digital health tools was conducted with the FCHVs (Figure 5.11). The assessment was done using a qualitative

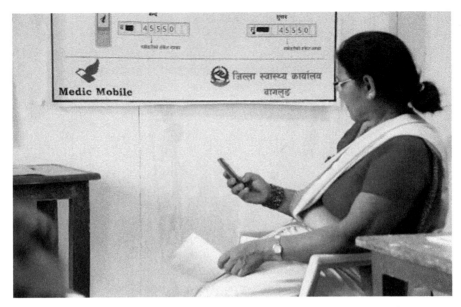

Figure 5.10 A female community health volunteer using Medic tools in Nepal.

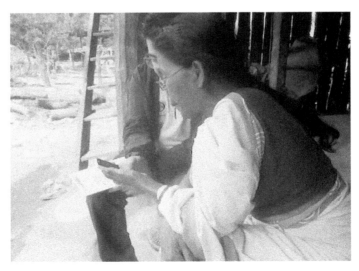

Figure 5.11 FCHV showing reminders she received for ANC visits of one of the pregnant women in her catchment during supervisory visit to her home.

approach to simply better understand the acceptability, perceptions of the training, and usability of the tools by the FCHVs.

The key themes listed in the following section were identified through preliminary data analysis, followed by coding of data around the identified themes.

Usability

CHVs perceive that the digital health tool is easy to use and navigate and that the tasks created remind them to follow up on individual clients. Additionally, the use of mobile phones has reduced their workload and the amount of time spent at the health post.

> After using a mobile phone I do most of the jobs at home and I don't have to go to health post several times to know about ANC period of pregnancy and not have to visit households frequently because everything I got on mobile phones and do most of the job at home and saves my time. I call to pregnant mother by phone for reminder and visit 1–2 time during her ANC checkup period after getting the reminder.
>
> **FCHV with physical disability**

Perceived Impact of Digital Tools on ANC Programmes

It was reported that these tools make it easier for health workers to prevent maternal deaths by immediately reporting the mother's healthcare needs and quickly responding with appropriate care as expressed by one FCHV: 'Earlier, we used to refer pregnant women to the health facility only if we met them by chance. But now, we get regular reminders and convey it to them. None of the pregnant women are missing now' (FCHV in Sindhuli of State #3). 'Many pregnant women do not come for antenatal check-ups in time. Before, we would call each of them from our personal mobiles. Now, we are happy that this mHealth tool is going to help us by sending the automatic reminders. This will save our time and cost of calling them frequently' (Incharge of Puja Health Post, Gaumukhi Municipality, Pyuthan).

Additionally, they reported that the mHealth programme helped identify maternal deaths, facilitating the rapid exploration of the circumstances of such events, enabling health system-wide responses.

Scale-up

The Ministry of Health leadership expressed a strong interest to scale up these digital tools and the government commitment to allocate resources for further implementation.

> After using Medic's tool in several districts, we realized the need to scale-up. This tool will help us build a health system that is accountable to the people. We from the Ministry facilitate an enabling ecosystem for mHealth, the local government allocates financial resources for implementation, and Medic provides the technology.

These elements together form a successful partnership model with potential to overcome the challenges of mHealth implementation.

(Shival Lal Sharma, Statistical Officer at Public Health Administration Monitoring and Evaluation Division, Ministry of Health and Population, informing elected members and health workers about mHealth and the CHT platform)

Conclusion

Community health system software can play a critical role supporting new models of care that make universal health coverage possible, enabling the equitable delivery of holistic and integrated services and the reduction of the financial costs of care for patients and for health systems. By adopting a HCD approach to training and supervision of CHWs it was possible to identify the training needs of the CHWs while having a deeper understanding of the contextual factors that are likely to influence design, uptake, and sustainability of the digital health interventions. By co-creating with the end-user, it was possible to identify training models that are suitable and sustainable to the context in which these digital health interventions are deployed.

The following recommendations are implied for training, education, and supervision of CHWs. Supportive supervision is considered best practice and usually contains elements of record reviews, observations, performance monitoring, constructive feedback, provider participation, problem solving, and focused education. In practice, supportive supervision strategies vary greatly in approach, content, and tools (Bosch-Capblanch & Garner, 2008), and there is little empirical evidence to help those implementing CHW programmes to design effective supervision systems that address the unique qualities that characterize CHW's roles in the community and the relationship to the health system. Providers and supervisors need to have the means to do their work; thus, poor drug supply, high staff turnover, busy clinics, and lack of supervisor transport reduced the impact of supervision. There is existing evidence on the disconnect between what we know about supervision and what happens in practice. For example, in a Zambian CHW programme, 50% of CHWs had no supervision (Stekelenburg et al., 2003) and even high-profile initiatives such as the Accelerated Strategy of Child Survival and Development (ASCSD) have reported inadequate supervision, with 38% of ASCSD CHWs in Mali having never been supervised and 81% reporting a lack of support (Perez et al., 2009), while in Malawi, 18–22 people made supervision visits to a given clinic giving inconsistent advice (Rohde, 2006). Getting supervision to happen is a challenge, and donors and national governments need to recognize this and support, fund, and manage supervision to ensure best practice is implemented.

With regard to use of digital health tools for supportive supervision, a key aspect of Medic's human-centred approach was the idea of using data to improve the process of face-to-face supervision, rather than using dashboard analytics to replace the role of supervisors. Some of the performance challenges faced by CHWs are more amenable through face-to-face interactions. There are also reduced opportunities for the few workers available to develop themselves by acquiring new skills through training and continuous professional development courses (Wasunna et al., 2008). Additionally, there is a need for better quality control of cascade training and this should be augmented with some simple measures of continuous education, dialogue, and supportive supervision.

Mobile phone technology could aid both the CHW and the community in communicating service needs and supply stock outs in advance, thus preparing the CHW's supervisor in the facility for the supplies that should be on hand before the CHWs make their group visit. Mobile phones can also be used by supervisors to provide on-the-job skills coaching for CHWs and by CHWs among themselves to enable them to support each other and ask questions when they encounter difficulties. As technologies become more readily available, approaches to learning and knowledge dissemination have leveraged on such digital innovations. E-learning platforms and courses are promising training and learning models given their unique advantages over traditional training approaches, such as increased accessibility to information, better content delivery, on-demand availability, self-pacing, and potentially reduced costs (Bhuasiri et al., 2012). However, successful e-learning relies on students having the knowledge and skills to use computers or mobile devices. While CHWs would benefit from the advantages of e-learning, it would not yet be feasible for them to effectively learn how to operate computers and programmes through distance e-learning. The majority of CHWs do not have access to a computer; they would be required to travel to an urban area to access a computer. Further, e-learning models may require interactive-voice response (IVR) technologies that have cost implications as these are expensive to maintain and eliminate the physical presence of the training facilitator and human interaction aspects of training. Therefore, a traditional classroom environment, where content is delivered through face-to-face interactions remains beneficial to the delivery of CHW training programmes in LMICs.

Acknowledgements

We are grateful to our Medic colleagues Nitin Bhandari, Dushala Adhikari, and Shreya Bhatt for contributing to the information presented in the case study. Special thanks to the FCHVS whose feedback on the usability of our digital health tools has been highlighted in this chapter. We also thank the Nepal Ministry of Health and Population representatives involved in the project for their continued support.

References

Agarwal, S., Perry, H.B., Long, L.A., & Labrique, A.B. (2015). Evidence on feasibility and effective use of mHealth strategies by frontline health workers in developing countries: Systematic review. *Tropical Medicine & International Health*, 20(8), 1003–1014.

Bhuasiri, W., Xaymoungkhoun, O., Zo, H., Rho, J.J., & Ciganek, A.P. (2012). Critical success factors for e-learning in developing countries: A comparative analysis between ICT experts and faculty. *Computers and Education*, 58, 843–855.

Bosch-Capblanch, X. & Garner, P. (2008). Primary health care supervision in developing countries. *Tropical Medicine and International Health*, 13, 369–383.

Chib, A., van Velthoven, M.H., & Car, J. (2015). mHealth adoption in low-resource environments: A review of the use of mobile healthcare in developing countries. *Journal of Health Communication*, 20, 4–34.

Feldacker, C., Murenje, V., Holeman, I., Xaba, S., Makunike-Chikwinya, B., Korir, M., et al. (2019). Reducing provider workload while preserving patient safety. *Journal of Acquired Immune Deficiency Syndromes*, 1(83), 16–23.

Freire, P. (2000). *Pedagogy of the Oppressed*. New York, Continuum.

Haines, A., Sanders, D., Lehmann, U., Rowe, A., Lawn, J., Jan, S., et al. (2007). Achieving child survival goals: Potential contribution of community health workers. *Lancet*, 369, 2121–2131.

Holeman, I. & Kane, D. (2019). Human-centered design for global health equity. *Information Technology for Development*, 26(3), 477–505.

Ilozumba, O., Dieleman, M., Kraamwinkel, N., Van Belle, S., Chaudoury, M., & Broerse, J.E.W. (2018). 'I am not telling. The mobile is telling': Factors influencing the outcomes of a community health worker mHealth intervention in India. *PLoS ONE*, 13(3), e0194927.

International Organization for Standardization (2010). *ISO 9241–210: Human-centered Design for Interactive Systems*. Geneva, International Organization for Standardization, pp. 1–40.

Jennings, L., Ong'ech, J., Simiyu, R., Sirengo, M., & Kassaye, S. (2013). Exploring the use of mobile phone technology for the enhancement of the prevention of mother-to-child transmission of HIV program in Nyanza, Kenya: A qualitative study. *BMC Public Health*, 13, 1131.

Jimoh, L., Pate, M.A., Lin, L., & Schulman, K.A. (2012). A model for the adoption of ICT by health workers in Africa. *International Journal of Medical Informatics*, 81, 773–781.

Kay, M., Santos, J., & Takane, M. (2011). mHealth: *New Horizons for Health Through Mobile Technologies: Second Global Survey on eHealth*. Geneva, World Health Organization, pp. 1–102.

Labrique, A.B., Vasudevan, L., Kochi, E., Fabricant, R., & Mehl, G. (2013). mHealth innovations as health system strengthening tools: 12 common applications and a visual framework. *Global Health: Science and Practice*, 1, 160–171.

Lester, R.T., Ritvo, P., Mills, E.J., Kariri, A., Karanja, S., Chung, M.H., et al. (2010). Effects of a mobile phone short message service on antiretroviral treatment adherence in Kenya (WelTel Kenya1): A randomised trial. *Lancet*, 37(9755), 1838–1845.

Mahmud, N., Rodriguez, J., & Nesbit, J. (2010). A text message-based intervention to bridge the healthcare communication gap in the rural developing world. *Technol Health Care*, 18(2), 137–144. doi:10.3233/THC-2010-0576. PMID: 20495253.

Ministry of Health, Nepal; New ERA; and ICF (2017). *2016 Nepal Demographic and Health Survey Key Findings*. Kathmandu, Nepal, Ministry of Health Nepal.

O'Donovan, J., O'Donovan, C., Kuhn, I., Sachs, S.E., & Winters, N. (2018). Ongoing training of community health workers in low-income and middle-income countries: A systematic scoping review of the literature. *BMJ Open*, 8, 10.

Palazuelos, D., Ellis, K., Im, D.D., Peckarsky, M., Schwarz, D., Farmer, D.B., et al. (2013). 5-SPICE: The application of an original framework for community health worker program design, quality improvement and research agenda setting. *Global Health Action*, 6, 19658.

Perez, F., Ba, H., Dastagire, S.G., & Altmann, M. (2009). The role of community health workers in improving child health programmes in Mali. *BMC International Health and Human Rights*, 9(1).

Pop-Eleches, C., Thirumurthy, H., Habyarimana, J.P., Zivin, J.G., Goldstein, M.P., de Walque, D., et al. (2011). Mobile phone technologies improve adherence to antiretroviral treatment in a resource-limited setting: A randomized controlled trial of text message reminders. *AIDS*, 25(6), 825–834.

Rohde, J. (2006). *Supportive Supervision to Improve Integrated Primary Health Care*; MSH Occasional Papers No. 2; Cambridge, MA, Management Sciences for Health (Google Scholar).

Sein, M.K., Henfridsson, O., Puran, S., Ross, M., & Lindgren, R. (2011). Action design research. *MIS Quarterly*, 13, 8–56.

Standing, H. & Chowdhury, A.M. (2008). Producing effective knowledge agents in a pluralistic environment: What future for CHWs? *Social Science and Medicine*, 66, 2096–2107.

Stekelenburg, J., Kyanamina, S.S., & Wolffers, I. (2003). Poor performance of CHWs in Kalabo District, Zambia. *Health Policy*, 65, 109–118.

Sudyumna, D.D. & Kitzmuller, M. (2017). *Climbing Higher: Toward a Middle-income Nepal (English)*. Washington, D.C., World Bank Group.

Wasunna, B., Zurovac, D., Goodman, C.A., & Snow, R.W. (2008). Why don't health workers prescribe ACT? A qualitative study of factors affecting the prescription of artemether-lumefantrine. *Malaria Journal*, 27, 29.

Winters, N., Langer, L., Nduku, P., Robson, J., O'Donovan, J., Maulik, P., et al. (2019). Using mobile technologies to support the training of community health workers in low-income and middle-income countries: Mapping the evidence. *BMJ Global Health*, 4(4), e001421.

6

Designing Pedagogically-Driven Approaches to Technology-Enhanced Learning for Community Health Workers

Shobhana Nagraj

Introduction

Training and supervision of community health workers (CHWs) has traditionally relied upon face-to-face methods of delivery. However, the landscape of training and supervision is changing. Improved mobile Internet connectivity worldwide, and the rise of affordable technologies, including low-cost mobile and smartphone devices (GSMA, 2019), have potential to transform the delivery of training and supervision to CHWs. Technology has been used with beneficial results in the training and supervision of CHWs through mobile Health (mHealth) platforms that: share clinical information and multimedia resources (Florez-Arango et al., 2011); provide real-time clinical decision support to support learning (Adepoju et al., 2017); provide remote supervision (Modi et al., 2019); and support the creation of professional networks through social media groups (Henry et al., 2016). Basic mobile phones can be used to provide training and supervision through interactive voice recognition (BBC Media Action, 2015; Amref, 2020) and SMS text messages (Zurovac et al., 2011; DeRenzi et al., 2012). Advances in technology have also enabled delivery of innovative and affordable training to learners worldwide using smartphone-based educational games, virtual reality, augmented reality, and massive open access online courses (MOOCs).

Technology-enhanced learning (TEL) is the use of technology to facilitate learning. Technology may be used exclusively, or in combination with more traditional face-to-face approaches (blended learning). Blended approaches to learning have been recommended for the training of CHWs (WHO, 2018), and may be particularly useful in low-resource settings, where access to face-to-face training and supervision is challenging (Mastellos et al., 2018). A core learning curriculum for CHWs has been proposed by the World Health Organization (World Health Organization, 2018), with potential for contextual adaption to meet

Shobhana Nagraj, *Designing Pedagogically-Driven Approaches to Technology-Enhanced Learning for Community Health Workers* In: *Training for Community Health*. Edited by: Anne Geniets, James O'Donovan, Laura Hakimi, and Niall Winters, Oxford University Press. © Oxford University Press 2021. DOI: 10.1093/oso/9780198866244.003.0006

the needs of local communities, and align with best practice guidelines for CHW training and supervision (Crigler et al., 2011). CHW training is now expanding to include pre-service training, with ongoing access to supportive supervision during their career course (World Health Organization, 2018). TEL may offer opportunities for innovative delivery of such programmes. Whilst the use of technology as the main or partial component of the learner experience has expanded over the last decade, there are few examples of how existing pedagogies have influenced the design and delivery of these novel approaches (Winters et al., 2018). Technology in the training and supervision of CHWs has potential to build upon existing pedagogical approaches to health professionals' education, whilst providing greater flexibility for the learner, teacher, and health system in which they function. This chapter presents a framework, outlining six key practical steps to consider when designing a pedagogically driven approach to technology use in the training and supervision of CHWs (see Box 6.1).

Why Is a Framework for the Design of TEL-Based Interventions Needed?

Approaches to the design, delivery, and evaluation of CHW training programmes are diverse (O'Donovan et al., 2018), making it difficult to compare existing training practices. There are also significant gaps in the evidence base for the use of technology in the training of CHWs (Winters et al., 2019). The lack of evidence for educational theory-informed TEL interventions for CHWs has limited our ability to understand the mechanisms by which CHW training programmes work, and the reasons why some fail to demonstrate effective learning (Winters et al., 2018). Frameworks to support the design of TEL interventions for CHWs can thus support the expansion of the currently limited evidence base, by providing a structure and context for design and evaluation of TEL interventions (Winters et al., 2018).

Identifying the Needs of the Key Players in the Health System

In addition, to the immediate communities in which CHWs work, there are other wider societal factors influencing their training and supervision. These factors include: *macro-level* influences such as government initiatives, guidelines, and targets, which may impact the content and methods of training delivery; *meso-level* factors, including the needs of the teacher/supervisor, infrastructure available for TEL, the technological ability of the teacher, and their knowledge, confidence, and familiarity

Box 6.1   Summary of the steps in designing a TEL-based training programme for CHWs

Steps in design of a training intervention and areas to consider

1. Identifying the needs of the key players in the health system
   Macro-level: The health system
   What are the health system's needs?
   - Understand the context of learning, the priorities of the government.
   - Ensure resources are available to deliver TEL, training, and supervision.
   - Ensure the training and supervision programmes are financially sustainable.

   Meso-level: The trainers/supervisors
   What are the teacher's needs?
   - Understand the motivations, challenges, and opportunities available for the teacher.
   - How is their time divided, do they have dedicated time for supervision and training of CHWs?

   Micro-level: The learners (CHWs)
   What are the learner's needs?
   - Understand the motivations and needs of the learners.
   - Decide how best to capture this information: for example participatory methods/qualitative study.

2. Integrate learner/teacher health system needs into shared learning outcomes
   - Decide how best to marry the needs of the health system, the teacher, and learner.
   - Use Bloom's taxonomy* to build a language for shared learning outcomes.

3. Consider how best to convey the information to learners
   - What learning theories will best support the subject area?
   - Which pedagogies will best support the delivery of educational content?

4. How can technology be used to best support learning and assessment?
   - How can learning theory be embedded into the technology?
   - How might TEL be designed to avoid cognitive overload in the learners?
   - How might TEL be used to encourage critical thinking?

5. **How can technology be used to support lifelong learning?**
   - What is the best way to make the learning interactive, engaging, and fun?
   - How can learning be embedded into the informal environment and/or the workplace?
   - Can design of the TEL help stimulate curiosity in the learner?

6. **What is the best educational environment to create for the training and supervision?**
   - Where will the training and supervision take place?
   - Who will be present?
   - Who will facilitate/lead?
   - Is the training best delivered in a small/large group or to individuals?

Bloom's taxonomy is a hierarchical ordering of cognitive skills.

with TEL; and *micro-level* factors of the learners (CHWs)—such as their learning style, access to mobile technology, demands on time, need for remuneration, and professional support. Negotiating the often varied, and conflicting, demands of these key players in the health system is important, both for the adoption and sustainability of TEL interventions, and to ensure that the needs of all players within the health system are met (see Figure 6.1).

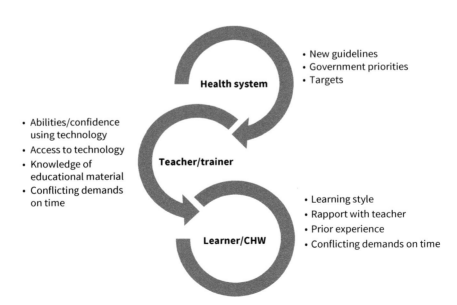

Figure 6.1 Factors affecting the needs of players within the health system.

Integrating Learner-Needs into Shared Learning Outcomes

A key step in planning TEL interventions for CHWs as a collective group, is an in-depth understanding of CHWs' motivations for learning. The motivations of CHWs to conduct their daily work are varied, and include both financial factors (e.g. adequate remuneration), as well as non-financial factors (prestige, career progression, and free health services for their families) (Abdel-All et al., 2019). Training opportunities can sometimes be viewed by CHWs as an additional burden to their already busy schedules, and might not always be their main priority (Abdel-All et al., 2019). Providing performance-based financial incentives for CHWs, may unintentionally lead to neglect of unpaid tasks (Kok et al., 2015). Understanding the motivations of CHWs, and integrating their training and supervisory requirements with their most important needs and priorities, is one way to support their learning, and ensure training and supervision are viewed as part of their work, rather than a luxury or a burden on their time.

Tip! Know your audience: explore the CHWs' motivations for doing their job, understand the challenges they face, their time commitments, and explore how best training and supervision can fit into their priorities and be integrated into their daily work.

It is equally important to capture the needs and motivations of teachers or supervisors delivering training to CHWs, to optimize the design of a TEL-based training intervention. One method to gain insights into the needs and motivations of learners and teachers, is through use of participatory approaches (see David Musoke in Chapter 8). Participatory approaches in the design of TEL-based training interventions use a non-hierarchical structure and democratic inclusion of key stakeholders in the design and delivery of training and assessment. Involving government officials, policymakers, CHW supervisors, and CHWs in the initial planning and throughout the design and delivery of TEL-based training has a number of advantages. Involvement of key stakeholders can: aid the dissemination of key government initiatives to the community-level; convey the needs and concerns of CHWs and their supervisors to policymakers; and resolve potential conflicts between key stakeholders in a timely manner.

Establishing shared learning outcomes that take into account the complexity of needs of the key players in the health system, is an important first step in the design of TEL-based training interventions. Learning outcomes are clear, measurable, and achievable statements that guide the knowledge and skills learners are expected to acquire during their training. Through involvement of key players within the health system in the design of learning outcomes, key performance and quality-indicators required by the government and policymakers might be more readily integrated with the learning needs of CHWs, ensuring a shared vision of CHW training within the wider health system.

Conveying the Information to Learners: Understanding How Adults Learn

Effective learning is the most important outcome of training and supervision. An understanding of how adults learn is key to designing and implementing training and supervision for CHWs. Unlike children, adult learners are required to take responsibility for their learning, and be self-directed in their approach (Merriam, 2001; Knowles, 2015). Adults bring their existing background knowledge and life experiences to new learning opportunities, and require that their learning is situated, meaningful, and useful to them. It is estimated that only a small proportion of adult learning is formal (delivered through formal means such as lectures and training days), and the majority of adult learning occurs informally or in the workplace (Swanick, 2005). In addition to providing formal learning content, TEL offers potential for informal learning opportunities through the use of social media groups, online forums (Gordon, 2014), and by creating more opportunities for reflection during workplace-based encounters with patients, through e-portfolios or remote supervisory support, including SMS-text messages delivered via mobile platforms.

Theories of adult learning or *andragogy*, may be useful when planning technology-driven solutions for CHW training and supervision, to best meet their needs, contextualize learning in their workplace, and co-create learning opportunities through the development of communities of practice (Wenger, 1999; Mann, 2011).

Embedding Learning Theory into Technology-Enhanced Learning: Finding the Right Fit

Theoretical frameworks of learning conceptualize how experiences of learning are assimilated, processed, retained, and built upon during the process of adult learning. These frameworks can be used to guide the design of TEL interventions. Embedding pedagogical approaches into the design of TEL interventions for CHWs not only provides clarity during the process of intervention development, but also provides a means by which researchers and policymakers can better understand and categorize *what* learning is happening, evaluate the mechanisms which lead to learning taking place, and establish *how* the learning outcomes for CHWs are met.

Technology-Enhanced Learning for Changing Community-Level CHW Behaviours

Behaviourist approaches to learning, focus on a model of 'stimulus and response', whereby a stimulus in the learning environment causes a change in behaviour of the learner (Merriam, 2001; Skinner, 2011). Behaviourist approaches in applied learning can result in standardization of responses, which may be useful in the context of quality and safety in healthcare. These approaches are often taken when the needs and demands of the health system, the political context, or government guidelines are implemented at the community level. An example would include embedding of standardized practices or checklists into healthcare (World Health Organization, 2009). Critiques of behaviourist approaches have challenged the importance given to the outcomes used to guide learning. In particular, *how* these outcomes are measured and *by whom* they are determined.

Behaviourist approaches may, however, offer potential to improve performance and knowledge of clinical guidelines, safety, and supervision checklists. Immediate feedback provided by a mobile phone or tablet, through reminder and recall systems, visual alerts, and sounds may alert a CHW to key information or areas of the checklist that require completion, or to any omissions that may have been made. Technology can be used in this fashion, to initiate behaviour change in the learner, working on a model of 'reward and punishment' resulting from the completion of a standardized guideline or checklist, until the guideline becomes embedded in practice.

This type of learning is potentially useful when the environment or context in which the CHW operates requires a certain standard of care to be implemented, such as a checklist for antenatal care or a vaccination schedule. Repetition of practice over time, leads to embedding of knowledge for the CHW. Disadvantages of this approach are that CHWs (being passive recipients of the learning), may only engage in superficial learning, and not fully appreciate the underlying reasoning for *why* the checklist questions are important to a patient or to their community. Whilst this may be helpful in situations when thinking may influence outcomes through the introduction of subjectivity, it can also lead to stagnation in the learning opportunities and personal growth of CHWs, and discourage clinical reasoning and a problem-solving approach. This may potentially impact CHW morale over time, if not met with positive reinforcements, such as incentives or rewards.

Learner-Centred Approaches to Technology-Enhanced Learning

Cognitive approaches to learning focus upon the processing of information by the learner and the formation of memories (Torre et al., 2006). The learner actively seeks to understand new information and relates this new information to previously formed memories (*schema*). Cognitive learning theory involves changes to the way in which information is processed (e.g. through repetition) and stored (organization of learning) by the learner, in addition to an outward change of behaviour. Cognitive approaches to learning for CHWs might involve providing a framework by which CHWs can link and categorize new information in relation to their life experiences, such as through the use of analogies, patient case studies, and anecdotes.

Technology can be used to embed cognitive approaches, by building new learning upon existing cognitive schema—otherwise known as *schema construction* (Piaget, 1952). Information may be presented to learners in increasing levels of difficulty, such as through a 'serious game', where a CHW might have to progress through increasingly complex and difficult scenarios. By presenting information in small chunks (*chunking*) and building upon existing frameworks of learning (*scaffolding*), the CHW will not get 'overloaded' with information (*cognitive overload*). In addition, technology can be creatively used by the CHW to set their own pace of learning, provide flexibility, and build upon existing knowledge. Instructional design (providing structure and meaning to learning material) is one method that can be used during the design phase of TEL approaches, to encourage schema construction, without causing cognitive overload (Gagne & Briggs, 1974). Cognitive overload refers to the amount of knowledge and sensory input the learner can process into their working memory (Young et al., 2014). If a learner is overloaded with information, their working memory and long-term memory and recall will be limited. Presenting information in small chunks and building upon existing knowledge (by understanding learner needs) is one way of ensuring cognitive overload does not occur. These factors can further be embedded into the design of TEL.

Supporting Lifelong Learning of Community Healthcare Workers and Critical Thinking

Constructivist models of learning recognize the importance of the previous experience of the learner, and build upon these experiences to construct new knowledge, often in a collaborative way (Torre et al., 2006). This model of learning is also learner-centred. As each individual CHW comes with their personal experiences and background, the way in which they interpret and create meaning from learning opportunities may differ. The CHW might start to challenge their previous model of the world and adjust their mental model of the world through learning in small groups and through creative use of patient case studies. This type of learning encourages problem solving and critical thinking, and requires the learner to take a more active approach in their learning, encouraging learning as a lifelong pursuit, rather than an activity limited to a training room.

A practical way in which constructivist learning can be embedded into TEL is through the formation of small groups for learning—such as participatory women's groups, and peer-assisted learning through online platforms, for example social media apps, or the creation of 'virtual teams' during online courses, and through the use of e-learning platforms. TEL may be used to provide learning materials or 'trigger material' to stimulate discussion before CHWs attend small group teaching.

An example of this might be TEL used to deliver pre-training content to the CHW through a 'flipped learning' model. Flipped learning is the use of a combination of TEL and face-to-face approaches (Gordon, 2014). For example, a CHW might be asked to watch a video online or to complete a questionnaire or pre-training quiz before attending face-to-face training. This will optimize time spent within the face-to-face environment, and build upon previous knowledge of the CHW.

Transforming and Challenging Previous Learning Using Technology

Transformative learning theory explores the learner's preconceived ideas of the world and challenges these assumptions of the world in order to trigger the learner to identify what they don't know (Mezirow, 1978; Taylor et al., 2013). The Johari window is often used to illustrate this process (Luft & Ingham, 1961) (see Table 6.1).

By challenging the learner through Socratic method (asking questions which stimulate co-operative argument and critical thinking), learners identify limits to their knowledge and view of the world. The learner is encouraged to critically reflect upon their preconceived ideas, challenge these ideas, and transform their perspective of the world. This form of learning may be very powerful, and creatively designed TEL can stimulate changes in world views through introducing new concepts. For example, by using evidence-based practices to highlight limitations to existing procedures; introducing narratives from people outside the CHW's direct community; and presenting a variety of views on one subject, in order to stimulate discussion, using media such as video, radio, photo-diaries, and documentaries.

Table 6.1 The Johari window

Open area:	Hidden area:
• known to self	• known to self
• known to others	• unknown to others
Blind spot:	Unknown:
• unknown to self	• unknown to self
• known to others	• unknown to others

Experiential Learning

The cycle of experiential learning by Kolb is used as one way of modelling how adults learn, and may be used as a framework for developing TEL interventions. Kolb's cycle of experiential learning involves concrete experience of a particular subject, followed by observation and reflection upon the experience (Kolb, 2014). From these observations and reflections, adults formalize concepts and make generalizations about the learning, and then test their findings out in practice (active experimentation). The cycle repeats as learners try out new experiences, reflect, and learn from these experiences (see Figure 6.2).

Kolb's conceptual model of adult learning, builds upon constructivist's theories of learning, whereby the prior knowledge and experience of an individual act as a foundation for creating learning opportunities between a new experience and building upon prior experiences. It may be particularly useful when designing TEL for the supportive supervision of CHWs, to guide CHWs through the cycle of experiential learning by observing their practice, reflecting upon their learning, and considering what they might do differently in the future.

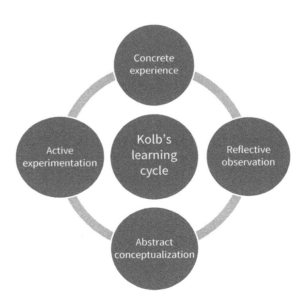

Figure 6.2 Kolb's cycle of experiential learning.
Source: Data from Kolb, D.A. 2014. Experiential learning: Experience as the source of learning and development. Upper Saddle River, FT Press.

Embedding Learning Within the Social Context: The Educational Environment

All of the pedagogical approaches explored in this chapter are implemented and embedded within a social context. Social theories of learning recognize the importance of the context of learning (the educational environment) and the community in which learning occurs (communities of practice) (Taylor et al., 2013). Learning and thinking are considered social activities, whereby learning is influenced by the environment and context in which the learning takes place. Social learning may be very powerful, in particular for groups of professionals such as CHWs, to encourage peer support and supervision. TEL interventions can be designed in a way to facilitate and promote a particular educational environment. For example, outdoor women's learning groups, might simulate a more informal environment compared to highly structured classroom-based learning. Considering the wider social context in which learning occurs is important, to decide which environment is most conducive to learning for a given group of CHWs.

Conclusion

TEL is a method of teaching delivery which may offer more flexibility to learners and teachers, particularly those working in environments where there are workforce constraints. Embedding pedagogical theory into TEL initiatives is important, and should be considered at an early stage during the design and implementation phases of training and supervision programmes. This chapter has outlined a six-step framework for approaching the design of TEL-based interventions for CHWs. Some examples of creative pedagogies for TEL have been presented, which build upon learning theory and take into account the social context of learning. The most important first step in designing a TEL training and supervision intervention is to understand the needs of the learners and marry these with the needs and capacities of the teachers and health system. This is best achieved by using participatory methods in design, including the principles of human-centred design, as discussed in this volume.

References

Abdel-All, M., Angell, B., Jan, S., Howell, M., Howard, K., Abimbola, S., et al. (2019). What do community health workers want? Findings of a discrete choice experiment among Accredited Social Health Activists (ASHAs) in India. *BMJ Global Health*, 4(3), e001509.

Adepoju, I.O., Albersen, B.J., De Brouwere, V., van Roosmalen, J., & Zweekhorst, M. (2017). mHealth for clinical decision-making in Sub-Saharan Africa: A scoping review. *JMIR mHealth and uHealth*, 5(3), e38.

Amref (2020). LEAP platform. Available from: https://amrefuk.org/what-we-do/projects/leap-the-mhealth-platform/

BBC Media Action (2015). How does the Mobile Kunji audio visual job aid support engagement between front line health workers and their beneficiaries in Bihar, India? Available from: http://downloads.bbc.co.uk/mediaaction/pdf/research-summaries/mobile-kunji-india-december-2015.pdf

Crigler, L., Hill, K., Furth, R., & Bjerregaard, D. (2011). *Community Health Worker Assessment and Improvement Matrix (CHW AIM): A Toolkit for Improving CHW Programs and Services*. Bethesda, MD, USAID.

DeRenzi, B., Findlater, L., Payne, J., Birnbaum, B., Mangilima, J., Parikh, T., et al. (2012.) *Improving Community Health Worker Performance Through Automated SMS*. Proceedings of the Fifth International Conference on Information and Communication Technologies and Development. ACM. 25–34.

Florez-Arango, J. F., Iyengar, M. S., Dunn, K., & Zhang, J. (2011). Performance factors of mobile rich media job aids for community health workers. *Journal of American Medical Informatics Association*, 18(2), 131–137.

Gagne, R.M. & Briggs, L.J. (1974). *Principles of Instructional Design*. New York, Holt, Rinehart & Winston.

Global System for Mobile Communication Association (GSMA) (2019). *The Mobile Economy, 2019*. Available from: https://www.gsma.com/mobileeconomy/

Gordon, N. (2014). *Flexible Pedagogies: Technology-Enhanced Learning*. York, Higher Education Academy.

Henry, J.V., Winters, N., Lakati, A., Oliver, M., Geniets, A., Mbae, S.M., et al. (2016). Enhancing the supervision of community health workers with WhatsApp mobile messaging: qualitative findings from 2 low-resource settings in Kenya. *Global Health: Science & Practice*, 4, 311–325.

Knowles, M.S., Holton, III E.F., & Swanson, R.A. (2015). *The Adult Learner* (Eighth edition). London, Routledge.

Kok, M.C., Dieleman, M., Taegtmeyer, M., Broerse, J.E., Kane, S.S., Ormel, H., et al. (2015). Which intervention design factors influence performance of community health workers in low- and middle-income countries? A systematic review. *Health Policy & Planning*, 30(9), 1207–1027.

Kolb, D.A. (2014). *Experiential Learning: Experience as the Source of Learning and Development*. Upper Saddle River, FT Press.

Luft, J. & Ingham, H. (1961). The Johari Window. *Human Relations Training News*, 5(1), 6–7.

Mann K.V. (2011). Theoretical perspectives in medical education: Past experience and future possibilities. *Medical Education*, 45(1), 60–68.

Mastellos, N., Tran, T., Dharmayat, K., Cecil, E., Lee, H.Y., Wong, C.C., et al. (2018). Training community healthcare workers on the use of information and communication technologies: A randomised controlled trial of traditional versus blended learning in Malawi, Africa. *BMC Medical Education*, 18(1), 61.

Merriam, S.B. (2001). Andragogy and self-directed learning: Pillars of adult learning theory. *New Directions for Adult and Continuing Education*, 89, 3–14.

Mezirow, J.E. (1978). Perspective transformation. *Adult Education*, 28, 100–110.

Modi, D., Dholakia, N., Gopalan, R., Venkatraman, S., Dave, K., Shah, S., et al. (2019). mHealth intervention 'ImTeCHO' to improve delivery of maternal, neonatal, and child care services—a cluster-randomized trial in tribal areas of Gujarat, India. *PLoS Medicine*, 16(10), e1002939.

O'Donovan J., O'Donovan C., Kuhn I., Sachs, S.E., & Winters, N. (2018). Ongoing training of community health workers in low-income and middle-income countries: A systematic scoping review of the literature. *BMJ Open*, 8, e021467.

Piaget, J. (1952). *The Origins of Intelligence in Children*. New York, International University Press.

Skinner, B.F. (2011). *About Behaviorism*. New York, Vintage.

Swanwick, T. (2005). Informal learning in postgraduate medical education: from cognitivism to 'culturism'. *Medical Education*, 39, 859–865.

Taylor, D.C. & Hamdy, H. (2013). Adult learning theories: Implications for learning and teaching in medical education. Web paper, *AMEE Guide* (83), e1561–1572.

Torre, D.M., Daley, B.J., Sebastian, J.L., & Elnicki, D.M. (2006). Overview of current learning theories for medical educators. *American Journal of Medicine*, 119, 903–907.

Wenger E. (1999). *Communities of Practice: Learning, Meaning, and Identity*. Cambridge, Cambridge University Press.

Winters, N., Langer, L., & Geniets, A. (2018). Scoping review assessing the evidence used to support the adoption of mobile health (mHealth) technologies for the education and training of community health workers (CHWs) in low-income and middle-income countries. *BMJ Open*, 8, e019827.

Winters, N., Langer, L., Nduku, P., Robson, J., O'Donovan, J., Maulik, P., et al. (2019). Using mobile technologies to support the training of community health workers in low-income and middle-income countries: Mapping the evidence. *BMJ Global Health*, 4, e001421.

World Health Organization (2009). *WHO guidelines for safe surgery: Safe Surgery Saves Lives*. Geneva, WHO.

World Health Organization (2018). *WHO Guideline on Health Policy and System Support to Optimize Community Health Worker Programmes*. Geneva, WHO.

Young, J.Q., van Merrienboer, J., & Durning, S. (2014). *AMEE Guide 86: Cognitive Load Theory: Implications for Medical Education*. Dundee, Association for Medical Education in Europe.

Zurovac, D., Sudoi, R.K., Akhwale, W.S., Ndiritu, M., Hamer, D.H., Rowe, A.K., et al. (2011). The effect of mobile phone text-message reminders on Kenyan health workers' adherence to malaria treatment guidelines: A cluster randomised trial. *Lancet*, 378, 795–803.

7
Mobile Phones and the Uses of Learning in a Training Intervention for Kenyan Community Health Workers

Jade Vu Henry

Introduction

Mobile phones are widely endorsed in the global health arena as an innovative and cost-effective vehicle for delivering educational content and providing supportive supervision to community health workers (CHWs) (Agarwal et al., 2016). In spite of this broad appeal, a recent review by Winters et al. reports that few mobile learning initiatives for CHWs are underpinned by educational research and theory (2018). The authors argue that most deployments adhere to over-simplified models of learning that fail to account for the complexities that emerge when new technologies are introduced into pedagogical practice. Building on their calls to incorporate more critical educational perspectives into the design, deployment, and evaluation of mobile learning projects for CHWs, this chapter will present some empirical and theoretical insights on how social relations of 'learning' are altered when training for CHWs becomes 'mobile'.

Background

The earliest scholarship in mobile learning involved the small-scale *de novo* prototyping of hand-held technologies to enhance and extend the activities of educational institutions in high-income nations (e.g. Sharples, 2000). In the course of refining the technical specifications for such devices, these foundational studies also made pedagogical and theoretical contributions. For example, research on mobile learning established the importance of accounting not just for the mobility of new technologies, but also for the mobility of learners as they 'moved' from one geographic space to another, across disciplines/domains of learning, through different formal and informal communities, at distinct and intermittent points in time (Kukulska-Hulme et al., 2009). It was argued that if new portable technologies were to support substantive

Jade Vu Henry, *Mobile Phones and the Uses of Learning in a Training Intervention for Kenyan Community Health Workers*
In: *Training for Community Health.* Edited by: Anne Geniets, James O'Donovan, Laura Hakimi, and Niall Winters,
Oxford University Press. © Oxford University Press 2021. DOI: 10.1093/oso/9780198866244.003.0007

innovations in teaching and learning, researchers and designers also had to consider the mobilities of learners and account for the emergent social practices that formed around such movements (Kakihara & Sorensen, 2002; Wali et al., 2008; Kukulska-Hulme et al., 2009).

Nearly two decades later, market-driven advances in mobile telephony hastened the widespread global uptake of robust, affordable, user-friendly, and pervasive devices, particularly in low and middle-income countries (LMICs) (Avgerou et al., 2016). These commercial innovations captured the attention of policymakers and funders charged with strengthening national health and education systems in these underserved regions (see World Bank and Independent Evaluation Group, 2011). In the perceived urgency to 'bridge the digital divide', research priorities for mobile learning shifted away from the foundational technological and theoretical endeavours of earlier years towards more applied interventions that could rapidly 'leverage' the features of the mobile phone to serve the global development agenda (Traxler, 2013). As a result, the mobilities of learners, as well as the unintended pedagogical and social changes brought about by the mobilities of new technologies, remain understudied.

To date, the prevailing approach to studying educational technology has instead focused on research questions related to 'what works?' This has generated positivist, instrumental studies to ascertain whether technologies have met prescribed educational objectives (Friesen, 2009). Experimental study designs have been favoured over other methodologies, while other forms of knowledge generated by practitioners remain ignored in favour of codified, standardized measures reflecting entrenched policy concerns (Oliver & Conole, 2003). Such research developments have led Selwyn and Facer (2013) to argue that the research in educational technology seems far more interested in what could or should happen than what actually does, observing that the ethico-political grounding of the Ed Tech domain has been shaped by the experiences and perspectives of powerful and vested interests, rarely showing any awareness of alternative experiences.

Purpose

In response, this chapter attempts to revisit and expand the theoretical and pedagogical insights established by early mobile learning scholars. More specifically, it will analyse what happens to 'learning' when training for CHWs becomes 'mobile'. It will argue that the movement of both mobile phones and CHWs raises important political questions about what it means to 'learn' when the training for CHWs 'moves'. The perspectives presented here sit within the disciplinary domain of Critical Educational Technology (Critical Ed Tech), an emerging field of scholarship seeking to: 'move away from a "means-end" way of thinking about how best to harness the presumed inherent educational potential of digital technology and... instead develop "context-rich" accounts of the often compromised and constrained social realities of technology use "on the ground" in educational settings' (Selwyn, 2010, p. 66).

As a contribution to the field of Critical Ed Tech research (cf. Eynon, 2018), this account aims to trace the social relations that formed during the design and deployment of a mobile learning technology for Kenyan CHWs, rather than to evaluate whether the academic research project achieved prescribed learning outcomes.

The insights offered in this chapter are understood as 'critical' in the sense that they scrutinize widely held assumptions about the role that mobile phones should play in educational projects for CHWs. Rather than producing evidence of whether set targets or objectives were accomplished by a mobile learning project, the study frame is broadened here, so that the targets and objectives themselves can be analysed in relation to other cultural, historical, and operational exigencies. The intent of this critical approach is not necessarily to dismantle dominant interests or undermine partisan agendas, but to instead: 'foreground attention to the way in which educational and emancipatory possibilities are realized and closed off, not in a future world, but through the choices and practices of educators, students, policymakers, and commercial companies in the messy realities of educational institutions today' (Selwyn & Facer, 2013, p. 12).

While policymakers and donors may favour impact assessments related to the *efficacy* and *efficiency* of educational technologies, Critical Ed Tech research opens up a different space to explore equally pressing concerns related to the *effectiveness* and *equity* of such interventions. As with the testing of healthcare initiatives (see Haynes, 1999), there are important questions about the effectiveness and equity of educational technologies that cannot be answered with randomized clinical trials and quasi-experimental designs, requiring instead observational methods and philosophical scholarship that capture the broader, community-related externalities and ethico-political dimensions of such projects.

Methodology

Research Context

The insights in this chapter are distilled from a doctoral thesis (Henry, 2018). Primary and secondary data for this research came from a larger three-year academic intervention known as 'the mCHW project' (http://www.mhealthpartners.org/projects/mchw). The aim of mCHW was to design, develop, deploy, and evaluate a 'pedagogically-rich' mobile learning intervention to train and supervise 90 Kenyan CHWs. The project emphasized participatory action research, practice-based learning, and iterative cycles of co-design, aligning itself with progressive educational theories and critical design methods. The mCHW project led to the production of a

smartphone-based tool to support CHWs in the assessment of childhood development milestones. The mobile learning intervention was deployed to 90 CHWs and
public health officers residing in the informal urban settlement of Kibera and in the
eastern rural village of Makueni.

The mCHW project was funded by the ESRC-DFID Joint Scheme for Poverty
Alleviation Research as a partnership between an established non-governmental organization) headquartered in Kenya, the University of Oxford, and UCL Institute of
Education where the author was pursuing a doctoral degree. The UK funding scheme
was viewed as a unique way of advancing more foundational social science in a domain that privileged applied research projects. ESRC would take the lead in addressing the 'world-class' and 'quality' aspects of social science research by promoting
theoretical and methodological rigour, while DFID attended to the applied aspects
of 'impact' and quantifiable 'progress' toward the Millennium Development Goals
(Scholz, 2012).

Methods

The ESRC-DFID joint scheme's emphasis on theory and research methods created
a rare opportunity to conduct a sociological investigation of how knowledge and
technological artefacts are generated in international development projects. The author acted as a participant observer of the mCHW project which was led by two doctoral supervisors. The insider-outsider doctoral engagement was meant to add a layer
of critical reflexivity to their work as principal investigators, and was a collective response to the funding councils' dual appeal 'to provide a more robust conceptual and
empirical basis for development and to enhance the quality and impact of social science research which contributes to the achievement of the Millennium Development
Goals' (ESRC & DFID, 2011, p. 2).

The study design for the research draws from canonical scholarship in STS by
Latour and Woolgar (1979). Their interdisciplinary academic work brought an-
thropological methods out of exotic locales and into the laboratories of scientific
institutions. In this anthropology of science, ethnographic accounts of laboratory
life trace how scientific facts and technological artefacts are produced through the
manipulation of equipment, data transformations, and rhetorical negotiations
(Sismondo, 2008). But whereas the scientific work in Latour and Woolgar's influential ethnography took place within the relatively contained walls of the Salk Institute
in California, the members of the mCHW project team were separated geographically, but connected digitally from numerous different settings in Makueni, Nairobi,
Oxford, and London. To study the dynamic, distributed, and digitally-mediated
work practices of this academic mobile learning intervention, the analysis therefore departed from classic genres of realist ethnography, adopting methodological
innovations in non-representational, multi-sited ethnography put forth by Marcus

(1995) and extended in Hine's later work on virtual and connective ethnography (2007; 2000).

Data Collection

Table 7.1 describes the primary and secondary data sources used for the analysis. Ethical approval for the research was granted from both the lead university and from the non-governmental partner organization. This approval ensured informed consent before data were collected, guarantees of confidentiality and anonymity for participants, as well as the right of participants to withdraw and have their data removed.

Table 7.1 Primary and secondary data sources for analysis of 'Laboratory Life' of mCHW mobile learning intervention

Data	Source	Date range	Description
On-line mCHW document repository	secondary	1 Oct 2013–June 2016	52 project documents, including funding call, research proposal, meeting minutes, and field reports
mCHW blog	secondary	11 Nov 2012–21 Jan 2016	49 blog entries
mCHW interview transcripts	secondary	29 Apr 2013–11 Dec 2014	282 pages of typed transcript from 31 baseline interviews with 10 CHWs, 5 public health officers, and 5 NGO administrators, and 2 community leaders
JH's field notes	primary	13–21 Mar 2016	42 pages of typed notes (from face-to-face contact with researchers, NGO employees, Ministry officials, and CHWs)
JH's audio files	primary	13–21 Mar 2016	10.5 hours of recordings (from face-to-face contact with researchers, NGO employees, Ministry officials, and CHWs)
mCHW photo-elicitation transcripts	primary	13–21 Mar 2016	66 typed pages of transcripts from 4 sessions with 10 CHWs and 5 public health officers
mCHW Twitter account	secondary	29 Nov 2012–18 Oct 2015	302 tweets/retweets
mCHW WhatsApp learning forum	secondary	19 Aug 2014–1 Mar 2015	1830 posts

Findings—CHWs, Mobile Phones, and the Uses of 'Learning'

Reflecting on the relationship between learning and mobile technologies, Enriquez has argued that, 'how we learn is not just an encounter of intellects mediated by tools, but a bumping into of bodies in spaces as part of ways of knowing in motion' (2011, p. 50). Drawing from concepts on the sociology of mobilities (Urry, 2000; Sheller & Urry, 2016) and of innovation (de Laet & Mol, 2000), she claims that when bodies and technologies move through physical and virtual space, 'what counts as learning' is assembled and reassembled as social relations evolve. Friesen makes a similar argument when he contends that definitions of learning and their attendant theories are themselves cultural artefacts which are shaped by technological, social, political, and historical patterns and contingencies (2013).

The following sections will describe how the mCHW intervention made training for CHWs 'move'. Using smartphones and a mobile learning application furnished by the project, CHWs engaged in learning practices that extended beyond the temporal and spatial confines of the formal classroom. These practices linked CHWs to other actors living and working in different geographic distances. The activities opened up new conversations for learning. Different groups of actors and materials were also integrated into their learning practices. In short, the mCHW project created novel physical and virtual places where CHWs engaged in continuous learning, implicating an array of additional people and material artefacts. However, these new spaces enacted and endorsed different 'ways of knowing' corresponding to competing theories and definitions of what it means to learn. When training moved, it raised new questions about the role of CHWs, their relations, and their responsibilities as learners.

Learning as Acquisition

Increased connectivity and the rising adoption of mobile phones worldwide brought great expectations among the agencies, ministries, and corporate organizations working to strengthen health systems in LMICs. A flurry of policy documents conveyed a great urgency to 'harness' these devices to supplement conventional classroom-based training for health workers in LMICs (e.g. United Nations ICT Task Force, 2005; Callan et al., 2011; Braun et al., 2013). The global health campaign to train one million CHWs in sub-Saharan Africa over the course of four years had been launched to address the lagging progress towards health-related Millennium Development Goals (see Earth Institute, 2011). A position paper issued by the Kenyan NGO partner of the mCHW project stated: 'Large-scale CHW systems require substantial increases in support for training, management, supervision and logistics… The CHW's most important tool should be his or her phone. The mobile phone can call the ambulance, get advice from a nurse in the clinic, or access a "smart" SMS system to retrieve patient information, get advice on drug doses, or log into a database on diagnostics' (AMREF Health Africa, n.d.). In this way, mobile phones were embraced as a 'solution' to overcome the barriers in implementing official classroom-based approaches to training.

CHWs were considered key players in one of several 'flagship projects' that made up Kenya's *Vision 2030*, a comprehensive government blueprint of economic, political, and social reforms directed at transforming the poverty-ridden nation into a middle-income economy (Oyore, 2010). A Ministry of Health policy document called the *Community Health Strategy* stipulated how these volunteer health workers were to support the fragile national health system as it struggled with the 'growing demand for care, in the face of deepening poverty and dwindling resources' (Ministry of Health 2006, p. 1). A 94-page training manual was developed by the Ministry of Health with the objective 'to build the capacity of CHWs to be able to lead their communities in health improvement initiatives in terms of disease prevention, health promotion, and simple curative care' (Ministry of Health 2007, p. 11). To officially initiate CHWs into their key role as 'lynchpins' between the formal health system and local community units (see Mireku et al., 2014), the Ministry training manual set forth a basic six-week course which was to take place in three different phases, each lasting two weeks. As shown in Table 7.2, there were seven different modules and a total of 31 sessions that correspond to the 'Level One Services' of the broader *Community Health Strategy*.

For each session, the training manual provided a description of the purpose, the learning objectives, materials, time frame, and rubrics. This basic face-to-face training was meant to prepare CHWs 'to gain the capacity to engage directly with households and communities to promote their health', and thereby 'sensitively and effectively add new knowledge and skills to those households and communities already have, building on and topping up this existing reservoir of experience' (Ministry of Health, 2007, p. 8).

Interviews with CHWs and other actors in the mCHW project highlighted the challenges of implementing this ambitious curriculum in resource-constrained environments. CHWs were convened in local churches, training rooms of NGOs, or community centres to receive the basic training delivered by different 'facilitators' from the Ministry or NGOs, who were recognized as experts in the topics of the various sessions. Absorbing the vast amounts of content during these face-to-face encounters proved difficult: 'I was not able to understand all the material that they wanted us to understand because they [the facilitators] were forced either to speed through some of the chapters because of the time and because they wanted to cover what they were told to [cover]' (CHW 1, Makueni, 8 May 2013, secondary data).

The CHWs were furnished with books, leaflets, and took written notes that could serve as references upon returning to work in community households. In cases where budgets for photocopying did not allow each CHW to take away their own set of reference material, copies were distributed to each zone and could be accessed by CHWs via the zone leader.

Table 7.2 Overview of course content for Kenyan CHWs

Phase 1 The community strategy (12 days)

Module 1 Concepts of health and development	Session 1.1: Health and development Session 1.2: Participatory methods Session 1.3: Leadership
Module 2 Community strategy for KEPH	Session 2.1: The KEPH at level 1 Session 2.2: Structures linking the community with the health system Session 2.3: Initiating the community strategy Session 2.4: Evidence-based planning Session 2.5: Organizing, registering, and mapping households
Module 3 Health promotion	Session 3.1: Introduction to effective communication Session 3.2: Adult learning Session 3.3: The key household healthy practices

Phase 2 Level 1 service provision (12 days)

Module 4 Mother and child health	Session 4.1: Pregnancy, childbirth, and the newborn Session 4.2: Community childcare Session 4.3: Caring for the sick child Session 4.4: Malaria Session 4.5: Diarrhoea Session 4.6: Measles
Module 5 Community nutrition	Session 5.1: Introduction to nutrition Session 5.2: Malnutrition
Module 6 STI, HIV/AIDS, and tuberculosis	Session 6.1: Transmission, prevention, and control of STIs and HIV/AIDS Session 6.2: Tuberculosis

Phase 3 Level 1 service provision and management (12 days)

Module 7 Water safety and sanitation and hygiene-related conditions	Session 7.1: Safe water management Session 7.2: Cholera Session 7.3: Worm infestations Session 7.4: Conjunctivitis
Module 8: Disability	Session 8.1: Disability Session 8.2: Rehabilitation
Module 9: Monitoring & evaluation	Session 9.1: Monitoring and evaluation Session 9.2: Reporting on community health status

---

Adapted From Linking Communities with the Health System: The Kenya Essential Package for Health at Level 1 A Manual for Training Community Health Workers, 2007.

The official training document envisioned that the basic course would take place over six weeks and be supplemented with refresher courses. It stated that 'CHW training should actually be lifelong, in fact, to strengthen them for their own lives as well as in their advisory role in the community' and accordingly allocated three days of continuing education per trimester, based on the priorities identified by the CHWs

(Ministry of Health, 2007, p. 12). However, refresher training was sporadic and subject to the vagaries of funding from international donor agencies. A Kenyan NGO worker explained:

> You are training 100 or 400 so you need a hall that can only be hired with money. The CHWs will not sit the whole day hungry and they will not come for training if there is nothing you are giving them because they have to feed their families at the end of the day. That is the challenge… It's a financial problem. You have to get the stationery, hire a hall, and give something for lunch. That is where the problem is. Competency is not a problem. The [facilitators] have the competency to train the CHWs. They have the manuals and all the information.
> **(NGO worker 1, 30 April 2013, secondary data).**

Budgeting aside, the administrative procedures and delays associated with this international funding also made it difficult to organize timely refresher courses that were immediately responsive to the needs of CHWs working in the field.

Mobile phones were seen by policymakers and practitioners as a solution to move the content of the official training manual beyond the spatial and temporal confines of face-to-face sessions. In the manner described by Labrique et al., they could be used: 'to provide continued training support to front-line and remote providers, through access to educational videos, informational messages, and interactive exercises that reinforce skills provided during in-person training. They also allow for continued clinical education and skills monitoring—for example, through quizzes and case-based learning' (2013, p. 166).

With mobile phones thus acting as vehicles for delivering content 'any time, any place', the spaces they created were extensions of the physical classroom, and learning was understood as a matter of receiving the right information in the right amounts, at the right time, in the right places. This widely endorsed, and relatively well-funded approach to mobile learning sought to 'move' the acquisition of concepts beyond the temporal and spatial confines of formal educational institutions and conventions. Resonating with behaviourist approaches as described by Friesen (2009), mobile phones were to serve as tools that promoted specific learning activities in support of health system strengthening, ensuring that as 'human resources for health', the 'CHWs practise within the limits of what they can achieve and for what they have been trained' (see Jaskiewicz & Tulenko, 2012, p. 4).

Learning as Conversation

In the ways described above, mobile phones could be used as vehicles to move learning so that the acquisition of information could take place out in new geographic and temporal spaces beyond the classroom. But early mobile learning scholars argued that such movement only promoted knowledge that was codified and simplistic; it failed to fully utilize the technical innovations of such new devices, nor did it acknowledge the agency of CHWs. Laurillard proposed that with sufficient time and resources for design, it would be possible to challenge digital technology to support more dialogic and reflective learning activities (2002). Drawing upon the Conversational Framework put forth by Laurillard (2002), Sharples demonstrated how mobile learning could involve not just the transfer of concepts across geographic and temporal spaces, but instead promote more sustained interactions between learners and teachers in a range of different settings and domains:

> Effective learning involves constructing an understanding, relating new experiences to existing knowledge... Central to this is conversation, with teachers, with other learners, with ourselves as we question our concepts, and with the world as we carry out experiments and explorations and interpret the results... And we become empowered as learners when we are in control of the process, actively pursuing knowledge rather than passively consuming it.
>
> **(Sharples, 2002, p. 506)**

In this light, the movement in mobile learning does not stop with the transfer of concepts from teacher and the remote learner. Instead, movement persists as concepts are iteratively built and elaborated in a 'pervasive conversational learning space' that enables 'continual conversation, with the external world and its artefacts, with oneself, and with other learners and teachers' (Sharples, 2002, pp. 508–509).

This dynamic notion of 'learning as conversation' and the Conversation Framework was cited in the original grant application to fund the mCHW project and shaped the initial design of the mobile learning intervention. Aligned with the approaches aiming to allow learners to control their pursuits of knowledge, CHWs were gathered for the initial participatory design workshop where they decided to use the mCHW project as an occasion to learn more about childhood development milestones. In response, the researchers looked to scientific expertise in public health and enlisted a survey known as the Malawi Development Assessment Tool (MDAT) (Gladstone et al., 2010) as educational content for a new mobile phone learning application. Just as certain computer programmes, theatre scripts, and political manifestos were thought to provide the impetus for specific thoughts, feelings, and/or behaviours among various sets of actors (Sharples, 2002), the MDAT would instantiate a mutual language that would enable the mobile phones, CHWs, and their supervisors to engage in conversation with one another.

The MDAT was an illustrated survey tool consisting of 136 items. Each item was a text phrase, often supported with illustrations, that prompted a researcher or health worker to ascertain a specific developmental milestone in a child, either by eliciting information from the parents, or by directly observing the child. An item corresponded to an isolated task or behaviour that was expected to be observed in a child of a certain age. The items were divided equally into four domains corresponding to the different areas of child development: gross motor, fine motor, language, and social.

Every domain was presented on its own separate A4 page in a grid format, with individual squares of the grid containing separate assessment items. Responses could then be compiled in a systematic manner to generate a global pass or fail determination of whether a child was progressing normally.

A developmental kit accompanied the MDAT survey instrument and was comprised of a small basket of props that were more suited to the local environment. This basket included 17 locally-appropriate, readily-available props, such as a pencil or ballpoint pen, string, dried maize, and Chitenje cloth. The user's manual was a 36-page document which provided a photo of the developmental kit and itemized the objects to be included in the basket. The user's manual offered guidance on how to administer the assessment tool, providing a brief description on how to ascertain each specific skill or behaviour in the child. There were also detailed instructions on how to score the MDAT to determine whether a child was progressing normally.

Because the MDAT was envisioned as diagnostic tool, concepts about child development were organized and presented to guide health workers during an encounter with a child. Loaded into the mobile phone in the form of a software application, the MDAT served two important pedagogical functions. First, it provided the concepts that the CHW would need to understand about child development: that child development is a multi-dimensional process involving gross motor skills, language and hearing skills, fine motor skills and visuo-perception, and social skills; that there is an age-related sequence of specific behaviours and skills associated with each of these different dimensions; that a child of a certain age is expected to hold his head up, grasp an object, sit up, etc. Second, it helped to materialize a 'task-practice environment for learners needs', laying out the specifications for 'experiential' learning exchanges that entailed 'acting on the world, experimenting and practicing on goal-oriented tasks' (Laurillard, 2009, p. 8). In this way, explicit concepts came bundled in forms of scientifically-validated protocol to promote experiential learning as CHWs interacted with children in community households in their service areas.

Sharples contends, 'to be able to engage in a productive conversation, all parties need access to a common external representation of the subject matter that allows them to identify and discuss topics' (2002, p. 507). Integrated into a series of interface screens on the mobile phone, the MDAT served as this common external representation, helping to create 'managed spaces for conversational learning' outside the classroom (Ibid., p. 510). For instance, a CHW who conducted an assessment of a child with the new mobile learning application could then retrieve this information to help initiate a dialogue with herself, engaging in self-reflection about what had happened during the administration of the health protocol: 'Was it easy to establish rapport with the child and the caregiver?' 'Were the props in the basket appropriate?' 'Did the assessment proceed smoothly?' 'What was the general health status of the child?'

These types of interrogations could then generate new understandings that informed a set of subsequent actions. For example, the CHW might then place a voice call that initiates a verbal conversation with her supervisor or a CHW peer. Another move might be to proceed to another screen where the CHW could register her level of agreement with the machine-generated assessment of the child's overall develop-mental status. Finally, the CHW might advance to a different interface screen and enter additional text describing her. All three possible moves leave additional digital traces of new 'learning actions' that assemble a text-based 'learning description' that the mobile phone automatically sends to the supervisors for feedback.

To further support these reflective learning actions digitally, the MDAT was coupled with a WhatsApp mobile messaging learning forum. Prior to this coupling, CHWs could utilize the comments fields of the new learning application to engage in text-based digital learning interactions with their supervisors, but they were not able to supplement this communication with photos or other media. The CHWs could resort to the generic SMS and voice features of the mobile phone in order to aug-ment their text messaging with other media or to communicate with their peers. But those SMS interactions and calls were subject to additional user fees, and the voice conversations did not leave behind substantial 'permanent marks' of those learning actions. In addition, the new mCHW application privileged one-to-one digital and voice interactions, and did not provide the capability to readily support group-based learning exchanges of interest to the researchers. Adding a WhatsApp learning forum as a component of the mCHW intervention supplemented the forms of conversation that had been made available through MDAT.

Embracing the constructivist pedagogical principles of the Conversation Framework, the mCHW intervention was designed to create a 'pervasive conversa-tional learning space' for mobile phones, and for CHWs and their supervisors to come to a shared understanding about childhood development milestones. This not only supported the movement of concepts across space and time, but also promoted a dy-namic form of knowledge production based on the iterative construction and refine-ment of concepts through experiential activities involving community households. 'Movement' did not stop after information passed from one geographic or temporal space to another, but persisted as CHWs engaged in continual dialogue with their mobile phones, supervisors, and peers during the course of their regular household visits in the community. Central to sustaining this form of cognitive motion was the agency of the CHWs in their role as learners. As Sharples has contended, 'Successful learning comes when the learner is in control of the activity, able to perform experi-ments, ask questions, and engage in collaborative argumentation' (2002, p. 508). By assembling the functionalities of the mobile phones with content of the MDAT, the mCHW intervention was designed to support and generate conversations between CHWs and their mobile devices, their supervisors, their peers, and between concepts and practices related to childhood development milestones.

Learning as Participation

This chapter has described how the mCHW intervention pushed the geographic and temporal boundaries of where and when the acquisition of concepts could take place. It has also suggested that this technology supported the creation of a new hybrid space, one where a shared language about common phenomena led to the iterative construction and refinement of concepts. This section describes how the mCHW intervention supported another form of movement, enacted not through the transfer of information or the dynamic conversations structured by the learning application, but through the unanticipated participation of a heterogeneous array of additional new actors from the local communities.

With the deployment of the mCHW learning application, the CHWs developed expertise in the assessment of child development milestones and gained the trust of increasing numbers of residents. The community had not always been receptive to the outreach services that were offered, and many CHWs felt the mCHW project added legitimacy to their identities as cadres of the formal health system: 'They [the community members] consider it [the phone] as something of importance. It's a kind of promotion to me as a CHW because... I used to visit them carrying books but now it is different... they are encouraging me with the phone... They are very happy also and some even seek to learn how the application works. They are appreciating' (CHW 5, 11 December 2014, secondary data).

One CHW suggested that the structured delivery of the MDAT's content via the phone application helped to streamline and fine tune his performances as a health provider:

> Using the tool? Actually it has made me feel... that I have that trust... because it has made my work easier, especially when I'm doing my assessments of child development milestones... It has [been] said that it [my work] is flowing. So it makes the parent from that particular household actually have that feeling this guy knows what he is doing; he is focused; he is going step by step.
>
> **(CHW 3, 16 March 2015, primary data)**

At first, the majority of children assessed by CHWs were found to be developing normally and did not require follow-up referrals to a local facility. This was consistent with the original objective of the new mobile learning application, which was to train CHWs in the early detection of childhood disability.

However, as the CHWs gained visibility in the community with the use of the new mobile learning application and their enhanced expertise, the mCHW research intervention began to enact unplanned performances—it started drawing out severely disabled children that had been hidden from the rest of the community. The mobile learning application functioned as an advocacy tool for disabled children. A CHW explains:

> As a neighbour, I've been there for so long, but I was not aware that this baby has disabilities. Serious. It took me a long time to understand that this baby has a disability because she [the mother] used to cover her, covering her from head [to toe] ... Nobody bothered about them [the disabled children]... We the CHWs, we

didn't know whether in our communities there were so many kids, because every mother used to close her kid in the house.

(CHW4, 16 March 2015, primary data)

Moving training for CHWs out of the classroom and across local households triggered a growing awareness among new actors about the unmet needs of disabled children in the community, creating a new social movement.

The mCHW learning application's 'script' or 'mutual language' for 'pervasive conversational learning' (Sharples, 2002) amongst mobile phones, CHWs, and their supervisors is now also supported by a dialogue with caregivers of severely disabled children. The CHW continued:

So to me, it was [before the mCHW project] it was difficult to start asking, 'Why are you covering your child from head to [toe]; the whole body; [carrying your child] on your back?' ... How will she talk about [this with] me? I told her, 'Now we are doing a new thing... We are assessing children on their growth; if they had failed in some developmental milestones; if they were born with some deformities; if they had any problems with their health.' So through the talk, she introduced her child... I am happy because [of] the introduction I brought to her and the information I brought to her. Now she is free and she is happy.

(CHW 4, 16 March 2015, primary data)

The mobile learning application provided CHWs with an occasion and set of talking points to initiate a dialogue with parents of disabled children.

In one study site, this growing awareness led to the formation of a new parent support group that devised a micro-credit scheme and an informal system of cooperative childcare:

So the mother told me, '... what you are doing and what you are talking, it is good'... And from that time, she allowed me to take photos and to bring anybody who was assistance to her house; but not a person who will come to her house and talk about her to create rumours and gossip. And since I assured her of that, everything has worked well. And now the team has grown to a big one. They were 15 mothers. Now she's recruiting another 20. The number is now 35... Even now, I know there are so many kids and what we also ask ourselves is why so many children within [the community] were born with cerebral palsy during this time.

(CHW 4, 16 March 2015, primary data)

In the other study site, a community forum was organized by a local school principal at the request of the CHWs. The principal invited one of the teachers, a mother of a disabled child, to present her story to the roughly 50 community residents in attendance. The principal proposed:

If it is possible to chip in, to come and work together to see whether we can introduce a facility, a small home. We have all this area. We have this land. We can have a small home where a teacher will take care of this child here all day and enable the mother to work for that same child. Because if they are bound like this, they will be bound forever. We are here to chip in for them and to empower them.

(20 March 2015, primary data)

Additional actors were thus assembled, including principals, teachers, elementary schools, as well as a proposed community facility for disabled students, and this would implicate different practices that included parent support groups, a variety of income-generating activities, as well as the manual fabrication of mud bricks by volunteers in the community.

The CHWs also developed paper-based patient registries to identify disabled children, to define their clinical and psychosocial needs, and to direct them to appropriate treatment and support from the formal health system. However, their referrals to Level 1 facilities led to reports of frustration and disappointment among parents who waited all day only to learn that local facilities were not staffed or equipped to care for their child. Because disabilities were not mentioned in the Millennium Development Goals, they were not explicitly addressed as a Level 1 service in the Kenya Community Health Strategy (see Ministry of Health, 2006). In a United Nations report, Groce contended:

There is a striking gap in the current MDGs: persons with disabilities, that is, the estimated one billion people worldwide who live with one or more physical, sensory, intellectual or mental health impairment are not mentioned in any of the 8 Goals or the attendant 21 Targets or 60 Indicators... The fact that persons with disabilities are not included in any of the MDGs and attendant Targets or Indicators represents a lost opportunity to address the pressing social, educational, health and economic concerns of millions of the world's more marginalized citizens.

(2011, p. 1)

Confronted with the immediate plight of vulnerable children, CHWs and their supervisors used the mobile phones to challenge the formal health system, rather than to advance their experiential training as public health cadres. They diverted their activities away from the priorities of the Community Health Strategy as they assumed the role of community activists working to forge new care pathways for the disabled children living in their communities.

In summary, when training for CHWs moved, new actors and materials were assembled in ways that supported learning well beyond the boundaries of the formal institution. Learning here was not about the individual acquisition or co-construction of officially-endorsed health-related concepts. It was instead an informal, emergent sociomaterial process by which many different repertoires of professional and lay expertise were assembled around a shared matter of *public concern* (cf. Latour, 2004). McGregor has argued that these kinds of social movements are constituted through a contingent process of 'collective learning' involving the formation of a collective identity, 'norms of social justice', a 'sense of solidarity', and 'knowledge pertaining to the mobilisation of material and cognitive resources' (2014, p. 221). Collective learning took place during the mCHW project in the form of 'experimental micro-political practices' that formed 'multiple loosely networked assemblages' (McGregor, 2014, p. 222) on behalf of disabled children in the community. With the mCHW intervention remaining open and receptive to the participation of a wide range of actors and materials, the practices of mobile learning shifted and expanded, resisting and subverting official training curricula and the technical specifications of design.

Conclusion—Mobile Learning and Moral Reckoning

What does it mean to 'learn' when training for CHW 'moves'? Global health researchers and practitioners have typically operationalized the 'movement' of mobile learning in terms of information transfer. Accordingly, mobile phones serve as vehicles to move concepts from one place to another according to the needs and demands of the CHW. In this context, educational interventions were often predicated on behaviourist learning theories and aimed to increase CHW access to curriculum-based health information. But the narrative in this chapter suggests that mobile learning generated additional forms of movement that lent themselves also to constructivist and practice-based accounts of learning. It illustrates how all of these definitions of learning—behaviourist, constructivist, practice-based—circulated through the lived experiences of CHWs as they encountered people and material resources affiliated with the formal health system, with the mCHW educational project, and with the local communities that they served. As Friesen argues, theories about learning were not so much a statement of biological or natural fact, but were social constructions that were intimately and materially connected to people, resources, and distinct disciplinary affiliations and policy priorities (2013).

In an empirical situation of resource scarcity, power asymmetries, and the exceptional mobilities of CHWs, mobile phones, and training practices, these competing definitions of what it meant to learn generated controversy and tension. This amalgam of learning theories and their attendant interventional approaches raised new questions about the role of CHWs, their relations to the formal health system and their motivations and responsibilities as learners—in ways resonating with Williamson's description of 'networked cosmopolitanism' in Ed Tech curricula:

Translated as pedagogy, networked cosmopolitanism promotes such a remixable mode of life through distributed learning, communities of practice, and the aerosolization of learning into the very atmosphere of digital culture. It shapes and sculpts a prospective identity that is individualist and self-interested yet also democratic and cosmopolitan in outlook; entrepreneurial and globally mobile yet also socially activist and locally committed; consumerist yet also countercultural; community focused yet also self-fashioning.

(2013)

Learning in this empirical case study was what Mol describes as 'multiple' (2002), enacted into the reality of CHWs' lives through conflicting power-laden arrays of people and cultural artefacts corresponding to distinct academically-derived theories.

As such, the controversies engendered by these varied enactments of learning could not be resolved with trials to determine whether or not mobile learning interventions were 'working'. If, as argued in this chapter, learning itself is presumed to be multiple, it is no longer useful to measure whether learning outcomes were achieved, or to even ask which learning theory represents reality. As Mol contends: 'If we can no longer find assurance by asking "is this knowledge true to its object?" it becomes all the more worthwhile to ask, "is this practice good for the subjects (human or otherwise) involved it?"' (2002, p. 165).

In the case of the mCHW project, the more salient issues for practitioners related to ethical and moral questions around, 'How to intervene?' or in Mol's words, 'What might it be good to do? What might the good be, here and now, in this case ...?' (2002, p. 169). This chapter supports Biesta's argument that education is a value-based rather than evidence-based practice, and that questions about the efficacy of educational actions are always secondary to questions of purpose (2010, p. 500). Accordingly, acting on the world requires not only scientific inquiry, but other forms of scholarship which attends deliberately and systematically to this question of goodness—to discerning the goodnesses that are enacted through the different sociomaterial arrangements that constitute learning in the challenging empirical terrain where CHWs live and work.

Acknowledgements

I am very grateful to all the co-participants of the mCHW project who so graciously shared their time and expertise during my field work. This work was supported in part by the ESRC-DFID Joint Scheme for Poverty Alleviation under Grant ES/J018619/2. Details of how to access the full mCHW project data set, consisting of the transcripts of 82 interviews with 24 CHWs, 9 of their supervisors, and 11 other public health professionals, exploring CHWs' roles and practices over the course of the design, introduction, and employment of the mobile learning intervention are provided on Oxford University Research Archive (Winters et al., 2015).

References

Agarwal, S., Rosenblum, L., Goldschmidt, T., Carras, M., Goal, N., & Labrique, A. (2016.) *Mobile Technology in Support of Frontline Health Workers: A Comprehensive Overview of the Landscape, Knowledge Gap and Future Directions*. Johns Hopkins University Global mHealth Initiative, Baltimore, Maryland, USA. Available from: https://chwcentral.org/resources/mobile-technology-in-support-of-frontline-health-workers/

AMREF Health Africa (n.d.). *Position Statement on Community Health Workers*. Available from: https://amref.org/position-statements/amref-health-africa-position-statement-on-community-health-workers/#gsc.tab=0

Avgerou, C., Hayes, N., & Rovere, R.L. (2016.) Growth in ICT uptake in developing countries: New users, new uses, new challenges. *Journal of Information Technology*, 31(4), 329–333. DOI:10.1057/s41265-016-0022-6.

Biesta, G.J. (2010). Why 'what works' still won't work: From evidence-based education to value-based education. *Studies in Philosophy and Education*, 29(5), 491–503. DOI:10.1007/s11217-010-9191-x.

Braun, R., Catalani, C., Wimbush, J., & Israelski, D. (2013). Community health workers and mobile technology: A systematic review of the literature. *PLoS ONE*, 8(6), e65772. DOI:10.1371/journal.pone.0065772.

Callan, P., Miller, R., Sithole, R., Daggett, M., & Altman, D. (2011). *mHealth Education: Harnessing the Mobile Revolution to Bridge the Health Education and Training Gap in Developing Countries*. iheed Institute, Cork, Ireland. Available from: https://issuu.com/iheed/docs/mhealthlearningreport

de Laet, M. & Mol, A. (2000). The Zimbabwe bush pump: Mechanics of a fluid technology. *Social Studies of Science*, 30(2), 225–263. DOI:10.1177/030631200030002002.

Earth Institute (2011). *One Million Community Health Workers*. Columbia University, New York. Available from: http://1millionhealthworkers.org/files/2013/01/1mCHW_TechnicalTaskForceReport.pdf

Enriquez, J.G. (2011). Tug-o-where: Situating mobilities of learning (t)here. *Learning, Media and Technology*, 36(1), 39–53. DOI:10.1080/17439884.2010.531022.

ESRC & DFID. 2011. *ESRC-DFID Joint Scheme for Research on International Development (Poverty Alleviation), Phase 2 Specification for Third Call for applications*.

Eynon, R. (2018). Into the mainstream: Where next for critical ed tech research?. *Learning, Media and Technology*, 43(3), 217–218. DOI:10.1080/17439884.2018.1506976

Friesen, N. (2009) *Re-thinking e-learning Research: Foundations, Methods, and Practices*. Peter Lang, New York.

Friesen, N. (2013). Educational technology and the 'new language of learning': Lineage and limitations. In: N. Selwyn & K. Facer (Eds). *The Politics of Education and Technology: Conflicts, Controversies, and Connections*. New York, Palgrave Macmillan, pp. 101–125.

Gladstone, M., Lancaster, G.A., Umar, E., Nyirenda, M., Kayira, E., van den Broek, N.R., et al. (2010). The Malawi Developmental Assessment Tool (MDAT): The creation, validation, and reliability of a tool to assess child development in rural African settings. *PLoS Medicine*, 7(5), e1000273.

Haynes, B. (1999). Can it work? Does it work? Is it worth it?: The testing of healthcare interventions is evolving. *British Medical Journal*, 319(7211), 652–653. DOI:10.1136/bmj.319.7211.652.

Henry, J.V. (2018). *Theorising the Design-reality Gap in ICTD: Matters of Care in Mobile Learning for Kenyan Community Health Workers*, PhD Thesis, UCL Institute of Education.

Hine, C. (2000). *Virtual Ethnography*. London, Sage.

Hine, C. (2007). Multi-sited ethnography as a middle range methodology for contemporary STS. *Science, Technology, and Human Values*, 32(6), 652–671.

Jaskiewicz, W. & Tulenko, K. (2012). Increasing community health worker productivity and effectiveness: A review of the influence of the work environment. *Human Resources for Health*, 10(1): 38. Available from: https://human-resources-health.biomedcentral.com/articles/10.1186/1478-4491-10-38.

Kakihara, M. & Sorensen, C. (2002). Mobility: An extended perspective. *Proceedings of the 35th Annual Hawaii International Conference on System Sciences*, 1756–1766.

Kukulska-Hulme, A., Sharples, M., Milrad, M., Arnedillo-Sanchez, I., & Vavoula, G. (2009). Innovation in mobile learning: A European perspective. *International Journal of Mobile and Blended Learning*, 1(1), 13–35. DOI:10.4018/jmbl.2009010102.

Latour, B. (2004). Why has critique run out of steam? From matters of fact to matters of concern. *Critical Inquiry*, 30(2), 225–248. DOI:10.1086/421123.

Latour, B. & Woolgar, S. (1979). *Laboratory Life: The Social Construction of Scientific Facts*. Beverly Hills, Sage.

Laurillard, D. (2002). Rethinking teaching for the knowledge society. *EDUCAUSE Review*, 37(1), 16–24. Available from: https://www.educause.edu/ir/library/pdf/ffpiu017.pdf

Laurillard, D. (2009). The pedagogical challenges to collaborative technologies. *International Journal of Computer-Supported Collaborative Learning*, 4(1), 5–20.

Marcus, G.E. (1995). Ethnography in/of the world system: The emergence of multi-sited ethnography. *Annual Review of Anthropology*, 24(1), 95–117. DOI:10.1146/annurev.an.24.100195.000523.

McGregor, C. (2014). From social movement learning to sociomaterial movement learning? Addressing the possibilities and limits of new materialism. *Studies in the Education of Adults*, 46(2) 211–227. DOI:10.1080/02660830.2014.11661667.

Ministry of Health (2006). Taking the Kenya Essential Package for Health to the community: A strategy for the delivery of Level One Services. In: *Reversing the Trends: The Second National Health Sector Strategic Plan of Kenya*. Nairobi, Health Sector Reform Secretariat of the Republic of Kenya.

Ministry of Health (2007). A manual for training community health workers. In: *Linking Communities with the Health System: The Kenya Essential Package for Health at Level 1*. Nairobi, Health Sector Reform Secretariat of the Republic of Kenya.

Mireku, M., Kiruki, M., McCollum, R., Taegtmeyer, M., De Koning, K., & Otiso, L. (2014). *Context-analysis: Close-to-community Health Service Providers in Kenya*. Nairobi, Reachout: Linking Communities and Health Systems. Available from: http://www.reachoutconsortium.org/media/1837/kenyacontextanalysisjul2014compressed.pdf.

Mol, A. (2002). *The Body Multiple: Ontology in Medical Practice*. North Carolina, Duke University Press.

Oliver, M. & Conole, G. (2003). Evidence-based practice and e-learning in higher education: Can we and should we? *Research Papers in Education*, 18(4), 385–397. DOI:10.1080/0267152032000176873.

Oyore, J.P. (2010). *Evaluation Report of the Community Health Strategy Implementation in Kenya* (Evaluation No. 2010/014). New York, UNICEF. Accessed from: http://www.unicef.org/evaldatabase/index_67793.html

Scholz, V. (2012). *Evaluation of the ESRC-DFID Joint Scheme for Research on International Development* (Final Report No. P2100057). Oxford, International NGO Training and Research Centre.

Selwyn, N. (2010). Looking beyond learning: Notes towards the critical study of educational technology. *Journal of Computer Assisted Learning*, 26(1), 65–73. DOI:10.1111/j.1365-2729.2009.00338.x.

Selwyn, N. & Facer, K. (2013). Introduction: The need for a politics of education and technology. In: N. Selwyn & K. Facer (Eds). *The Politics of Education and Technology: Conflicts, Controversies, and Connections*. New York, Palgrave Macmillan, pp. 1–17.

Sharples, M. (2000). The design of personal mobile technologies for lifelong learning. *Computers and Education*, 34(3), 177–193. DOI:10.1016/S0360-1315(99)00044-5.

Sharples, M. (2002). Disruptive devices: Mobile technology for conversational learning. *International Journal of Continuing Engineering Education and Life Long Learning*, 12(5–6), 504–520. DOI:10.1504/IJCEELL.2002.002148.

Sheller, M. & Urry, J. (2016). The new mobilities paradigm. *Environment and Planning A*, 38, 207–226. DOI:10.1068/a37268.

Sismondo, S. (2008). Science and technology studies and an engaged program. In: E.J. Hackett, O. Amsterdamska, M. Lynch, & J. Wajcman (Eds). *The Handbook of Science and Technology Studies* (Third Edition). Cambridge MA, MIT Press.

Traxler, J. (2013). mLearning solutions for international development: Rethinking the thinking. *Digital Culture and Education*, 5 (2), 74–85. Available from: http://www.digitalcultureandeducation.com/cms/wp-content/uploads/2013/12/traxler.pdf

United Nations ICT Task Force (2005). Harnessing the potential of ICT for education: A multistakeholder approach. *Proceedings from the Dublin Global Forum of the United Nations ICT Task Force*. United Nations Publications, New York. Available from: https://digitallibrary.un.org/record/561571?ln=fr

Urry, J. (2000). Mobile sociology. *The British Journal of Sociology*, 51(1), 185–203. DOI:10.1111/j.1468-4446.2009.01249.x.

Wali, E., Winters, N., & Oliver, M. (2008). Maintaining, changing and crossing contexts: An activity theoretic reinterpretation of mobile learning. *Research in Learning Technology*, 16(1), DOI:10.3402/rlt.v16i1.10884.

Williamson, B. (2013). Networked cosmopolitanism? Shaping learners by remaking the curriculum of the future. In: N. Selwyn & K. Facer (Eds). *The Politics of Education and Technology: Conflicts, Controversies, and Connections*. New York, Palgrave Macmillan, pp. 39–59.

Winters, N., Oliver, M., Mukami, D., Lakati, A., Mbae, S., Wanjiru, H., et al. (2015). mCHW: A mobile learning intervention for community health workers. University of Oxford, UK. Available from: https://ora.ox.ac.uk/objects/uuid:08b9f5e2-b677-4142-ade7-87603ab1533f

Winters, N., Langer, L., & Geniets, A. (2018). Scoping review assessing the evidence used to support the adoption of mobile health (mHealth) technologies for the education and training of community health workers (CHWs) in low-income and middle-income countries. *BMJ Open*, 8(7), e019827. DOI:10.1136/bmjopen-2017-019827.

World Bank & Independent Evaluation Group (2011). *Capturing Technology for Development: An Evaluation of World Bank Group Activities in Information and Communication Technologies*. Washington DC. Available from: http://hdl.handle.net/10986/2370

8
Using Participatory Approaches for Community Health Worker Training

David Musoke

Introduction

Community health workers (CHWs) continue to play an important role in supporting health systems, particularly in low and middle-income countries (LMICs), and training is an increasingly crucial component of CHW programmes. Training CHWs serves to enhance their knowledge, skills, and capabilities, hence contributing to an overall improvement in their performance (WHO, 2018). As opposed to more traditional training approaches, in which learners are seen as passive 'recipients' of knowledge, participatory approaches ensure that learners are actively involved in the educational process. From this perspective, learning can be understood as a continuing process of 'participation' rather than a discrete instance of knowledge 'acquisition' (Sfard, 1998).

Inspired by Freire's *Pedagogy of the Oppressed* (1968), which encouraged oppressed communities to examine the structural mechanisms perpetuating their oppression (and which argued that knowledge can serve to reinforce the position of the powerful in society), participatory approaches aim to reduce inequities between trainers and trainees (Baum et al., 2006). Learners are positioned as creative and capable participants in a process of dialogue, reflection, and action, while trainers have a role as catalysts and facilitators (Pretty et al., 1995). Through participatory processes, local and individual experience is understood as a legitimate and important form of knowledge.

Accordingly, participatory approaches examine the knowledge, values, needs, experiences, skills, and orientation of learners, in the context of their cultural, historical, social, and economic situations. Benefits of using participatory approaches in training include building teamwork among learners, learning from people's experiences, building confidence, enhancing critical thinking, and making the learning process more relevant and interesting (PRIA, 2013). Learners who have undergone participatory training can feel a sense of ownership of the knowledge generated, as well as a sense of empowerment to take action, which in turn can lead to positive and long-lasting changes in practice (Hill-Briggs et al., 2007).

David Musoke, *Using Participatory Approaches for Community Health Worker Training* In: *Training for Community Health*.
Edited by: Anne Geniets, James O'Donovan, Laura Hakimi, and Niall Winters, Oxford University Press.
© Oxford University Press 2021. DOI: 10.1093/oso/9780198866244.003.0008

This chapter explores key elements of the use of participatory methods in training of CHWs, including ensuring active engagement of participants in the learning process and facilitating shared experiences, thus helping make training more responsive to their needs as learners. In addition, training should provide opportunities for close interaction between trainees and facilitators, generation of ideas, and problem-solving. Participatory training should consider the needs of participants, provide an environment where learners feel comfortable, as well as facilitate peer-to-peer learning. The need for a combination of visual, written, and hands-on methods to facilitate participatory learning of CHWs is also presented. The participatory training methods discussed in this chapter include role-plays, demonstrations, songs, small and large group discussions, brainstorming, debates, simulations, exercises, field trips, gallery walks, class presentations, practicals, case studies, and interactive exercises. This chapter then seeks to evaluate the relative advantages and disadvantages of each method, and highlights the importance of local contextual factors in selecting appropriate participatory approaches in CHW training programmes.

Role-Plays

Role-plays involve a group of people acting out roles to depict real-world scenarios (Stokoe, 2011). Such role-plays have been recommended for use in training of CHWs (CDC, 2009), particularly for difficult or unfamiliar scenarios. Role-plays are useful in improving communication among trainees, as well as effective and enjoyable when well planned (Ments, 1999). After identifying a situation of concern and providing information about it to the trainees, roles to be acted should be assigned. CHWs need to be knowledgeable and comfortable with the assigned roles for the success of the activity. Sometimes, the facilitator may need to provide trainees with a demonstration of how the role-play should be conducted before beginning the session. Once the CHWs have understood their roles, they should act out the scenario in front of the entire group. It is important that the CHWs who are not actively involved in the role-play take note of the emerging issues and learning during the activity, so that these may be discussed later in a group setting.

After the role-play has been conducted, the facilitator helps the participants to provide feedback from the activity, with a focus on asking questions and obtaining clarifications. This feedback can help to improve future role-play activities, as well as aiding the facilitator to assess whether key messages from the role-play have been identified by the CHWs. This assessment can be done by asking questions to the participants or requesting them to write a summary of their learning. The method of feedback after the role-play (either written or oral) should be appropriate for the setting and decided in a participatory manner.

In training sessions where CHWs need to learn about various scenarios, different CHWs should be involved in subsequent role-plays, in order to ensure everyone has an opportunity to participate. As an example, role-plays could be used effectively in the training of CHWs to carry out household visiting (Millennium Villages Project, 2013). In this scenario, a CHW would approach a household member to carry out a particular health activity, such as the immunization of a child. One trainee would take on the role of a 'CHW', while another would be the 'household member'. Both individuals would need to be oriented on their roles by the facilitator before the activity. For example, the 'CHW' would need to understand the intended purpose of the visit to the household, while the 'household member' could be asked to depict a difficult scenario for the 'CHW'. As an example, the 'household member' may be asked to have strong reasons for disliking immunization for their children. Such a role-play would demonstrate to the trainees how CHWs can approach a community member and deal with such as a scenario to convince them of the importance of child immunization. Role-plays can also be used as a precursor to other approaches, such as brainstorming or group work. For example, after the role-play on household visiting, a group discussion could be held on ways in which CHWs can enhance community members' uptake of public health interventions in their area.

Demonstrations

Demonstrations can be used during training of CHWs to provide a practical illustration of a task or technique. Demonstrations are useful in a session that requires trainees to observe an activity being carried out to enhance their learning. Demonstrations as a form of observational learning not only enhance acquisition of skills but also support the use of the acquired knowledge in real life (Mohan, 2010). In addition, demonstrations improve understanding of complex skills and techniques among trainees (Basheer et al., 2017), as well as enhancing practical tasks. For example, during the training of CHWs on home management of diarrhoea, a demonstration on preparation of oral rehydration salts (ORS) could be done. This activity would require the facilitator to have all the necessary supplies for the demonstration prepared in advance. After the demonstration, a discussion should provide trainees with the opportunity to ask questions and seek clarification, so as to avoid unidirectional flow of information. It is important that the facilitator has sufficient knowledge of the subject in order to ensure proper conduct of the demonstration, as well as being able to respond to any emerging questions. Use of commentary during the demonstrations ensures trainees benefit from both visual and verbal modes of communication. Utilization of both visual and audio senses in a training activity is expected to engage participants more and further enhance learning (Rasul et al., 2011). Where resources permit, CHWs can attempt to replicate the demonstration themselves as a form of participatory learning. This helps the facilitator to assess the performance of the trainees, and provide further guidance on carrying out the task. Given that CHWs participating in the training need to observe the demonstration, the method may not be suitable for large groups. Therefore, demonstrations may better suit facilitating small-group learning as a form of participatory training.

Songs

Songs can be used as a participatory method during training of CHWs. In addition to enhancing the learning process, use of songs in training can be fun for participants (Kuśnierek, 2016), making the experience memorable. Although songs have extensively been used among children, they have not been used a lot among CHWs. Therefore, there is potential to incorporate songs in the training of CHWs as a participatory approach. The use of songs can be particularly useful while training CHWs who have low literacy levels (Van Boetzelaer et al., 2019). Indeed, songs can be appropriate when other traditional methods such as lectures may not be possible. As part of the training, CHWs can be requested to compose songs on particular topics of interest. Otherwise, the facilitator may introduce pre-composed songs, and teach the CHWs how to sing them. Giving CHWs the opportunity to compose their own songs gives them the opportunity to show creativity and initiative in the learning process. The benefits of using songs in training CHWs can be two-fold. First of all, songs can help CHWs appreciate the subject being taught. For example, a song on maternal health regarding the importance of antenatal care (ANC) could be useful to understand the significance of the practice. Such a song could highlight the benefits of attending ANC as well as the negative outcomes that could result if pregnant women fail to attend. Training of CHWs using songs, among other methods, has been carried out for maternal, newborn, and child health activities (Health Child Uganda, 2015).

Second, the use of songs in training also empowers CHWs to use them while carrying out health communication in communities during their practice. Indeed, songs can be an effective way to communicate health messages, particularly to rural communities in LMICs (Naugle & Hornik, 2014). Use of songs in health promotion is not only informative but also enjoyable to the audience. However, the facilitator would need to have experience in the use of songs in training so as to adequately provide guidance to CHWs both in composition and delivery. In situations where the facilitator has limited expertise in music, an individual with more knowledge and skills may be invited to support this component of the training.

Small and Large Group Discussions

Group discussions can effectively engage CHWs during their training. Such discussions would ensure the CHWs take an active part in the learning, as well as benefiting from each other's knowledge. Discussions also facilitate the sharing of experiences among CHWs, which makes an important addition to the expertise of the facilitator. During training, the facilitator would need to introduce the topic of discussion, and to ensure trainees clearly understand it. It is ideal that the trainees are given an opportunity to ask questions and seek clarification before the group work commences. After the introductory session, the facilitator then forms the groups for discussion.

Depending on the topic of discussion, the groups can be heterogeneous or homogeneous. Indeed, if the subject of interest is on an issue that would not require diversity among participants, then a homogeneous group could be selected. For example, if the training is on a gender issue in which both males and females may not openly express themselves if together, then gender specific groups could be considered. Otherwise, a group with both males and females would be ideal to discuss most health issues.

In addition to gender, other socio-demographic characteristics of the trainees could be considered during formulation of groups, such as age, marital status, level of education, economic status, and religion. Having a diverse group ensures that different perspectives and experiences from trainees are explored during the discussion. Small groups (5–10 people) are normally preferred as they enhance teamwork, arouse trainee interest, and support self-directed learning (Meo, 2013). A large group, by contrast, could mean some trainers are not able to make substantial contributions to the discussion.

It is important that each group has a chairperson (who could be one of the trainees or a facilitator) and a rapporteur. The chairperson would moderate the conduct of the discussion and ensure it goes on as planned. The role of the rapporteur would be to take notes on the content of the discussion that can later be presented to the entire group of participants. Ideally, once all the groups have completed their discussion, a plenary session including all trainees should take place. This plenary session would be used for every group to present key issues from their discussion, and to listen to feedback from the entire group. The plenary session provides an important opportunity for trainees to consider issues raised in other groups.

Brainstorming

Brainstorming is another method that can be used to facilitate participatory learning among CHWs. This method can be used when the trainees can share ideas or experiences related to a particular topic (Smartsheet, 2019). In addition, brainstorming can be useful when the facilitator wishes to actively involve the trainees in the generation of knowledge (Gogus, 2013). During brainstorming, the facilitator introduces a topic to the trainees, then asks them to make contributions to it in a spontaneous, uninhibited manner. It is important to stress to the CHWs early on that there are no incorrect answers, and that all contributions are valid, so as to allay any fears of providing 'wrong' answers. The facilitator should also endeavour to ensure that as many CHWs as possible take an active part in the brainstorming session, rather than allowing a few individuals to dominate. To achieve this, a facilitator could ask for contributions from specific trainees, or give opportunities to those who may not have said anything.

After the brainstorming is complete, it is important for the facilitator to summarize key emerging issues, and present them to the trainees. Summarizing the emerging themes ensures that the CHWs are reminded of the important messages for their future use. Brainstorming can be used as a stand-alone approach, or as a precursor to another method such as a lecture or group discussion. Brainstorming can also be helpful to the facilitator to assess the level of knowledge of trainees on a subject, which can in turn inform other aspects of the training. Indeed, after a brainstorming session, a facilitator can decide how best to approach the training having established the level of knowledge of the trainees.

Debates

A debate is a discussion that normally involves two sides, one in favour of and the other opposing a topic of interest. Although debates have primarily been used in public meetings, legislative assemblies, and training institutions including schools and universities (Wikipedia, 2019), they can support participatory training of CHWs. Debates can be used in training on a topic that is complex or controversial, or when views for and against a subject are required to be explored among trainees (Fournier-Sylvester, 2013). The two groups should be aware of the task at hand, and told their specific role in the debate in advance to ensure they prepare adequately. This may include the trainees conducting some research. The facilitator (often called a moderator) introduces the topic to the trainees, and provides guidelines to be followed during the debate. The two groups are given an opportunity to present their views on the topic, sometimes opening the discussion to other participants at a later stage. The participants can make their own contribution to the topic, or address questions to the two groups for clarity or more information. The facilitator needs to ensure both groups are given adequate opportunity to support or oppose the topic of the debate (which is sometimes called a motion).

Although some forms of debate conclude with an outcome of the contest (which could be decided by the audience or judges), this is not normally the case during a training. Indeed, after a discussion following a debate in a training, the facilitator needs to summarize the key points, and provide the takeaway message to trainees. Although debates can be used as a separate method for training CHWs, they may also be used as a precursor to other forms of training. For example, after a debate a facilitator may go ahead and make a presentation to the CHWs on the subject of interest. Debates can enhance public speaking of trainees, facilitate deeper understanding of issues, and promote research. In addition, debates stimulate thinking and engage trainees in an intellectual manner. However, debates may not be suited to learners with low levels of education, who may find the method complex.

Simulations

Simulations involve learning through guided, interactive reconstructions of real-life experiences. Although such simulations have mainly been used in the military and aviation fields, they are increasingly being used in health and medicine (Lateef, 2010).

Such a technique can be used when equipment or technology is not readily available during the training, or when the actual situation of interest cannot be used. For example, while training CHWs on a new facility for handwashing yet to be obtained for actual demonstration, a simulation can be employed. In addition, simulations can be used when training CHWs in certain clinical procedures such as administering treatment that cannot be done on actual patients. Simulations help to protect patients from unnecessary risks, yet allow trainees to gain the knowledge, skills, and attitudes needed for their work (Aggarwal et al., 2010). For this reason, simulation-based training addresses ethical issues as well as practical concerns, especially regarding patients.

Use of simulations in training CHWs gives them hands-on experience in the subject of interest, making them better prepared for performance of the task as part of their future practice. During the simulation, CHWs can use realistic scenarios, techniques, or equipment for several times until they master the procedure. This repeated exposure makes CHWs more prepared to face real-life situations during their work. In addition to the training itself, simulations can be used to test the proficiency of CHWs in performing certain tasks, which is a significant advantage in using the method. If used as part of team training, simulations also enhance interpersonal communication, which is critical in performing certain tasks such as outbreak investigation. After a simulation exercise, it is important to have a debriefing session with the trainees to get feedback on the process and any concerns they may have. It is important to note that simulations of some technology or procedures may not always be available or possible, which may limit their use in certain circumstances.

Exercises

Exercises can be incorporated into training of CHWs to enhance their participation and facilitate learning. Such exercises can be given after a training session has been completed, for example following a lecture. The exercise, which can be individual or for a group, would require the CHWs to undertake it, and report to the facilitator. Group exercises can be useful, especially for a large number of training participants. However, active involvement of all members in a group cannot always be guaranteed, which presents an important limitation. Depending on the training, the exercise can be written, oral, practical, or a combination of methods. Exercises can particularly be helpful when a facilitator wishes to confirm mastery of a subject by trainees (Špernjak & Šorgo, 2018) before they use the knowledge or skill in their work. Exercises also foster experiential learning, as participants are actively involved in a task. In addition, participants of training involving exercises are normally motivated and develop interactive skills during the process, which is key in participatory learning. As an example, CHWs can be given an exercise to list household practices that contribute to faecal-oral diseases. After the exercise, it is important that the facilitator provides feedback to the participants to ensure they learn from the process, and thus improve their knowledge and skills. It should be noted that providing individual feedback in training that involves many participants could be challenging to the facilitator. In addition, CHWs can become frustrated if they fail the exercise, which could affect their involvement in other training activities.

It is for this reason that some facilitators may decide not to grade the exercise, or provide marks to the trainees. However, other facilitators may prefer disclosing performance to trainees so that those who have performed well are inspired and sometimes rewarded. Trainees who may not have performed well in a certain exercise could also work harder in the next one if they are aware of the reward that comes with doing well. Therefore, the use of exercises needs to be carefully considered during training of CHWs, paying consideration to what best suits the learners.

Field Trips

Field trips can be used as a form a participatory training of CHWs. Such field trips can be a stand-alone training method or used in combination with other approaches. Field trips are especially appropriate when the topic of the training can best be appreciated through exposure at a field site (Myers & Jones, 2003). For example, if CHWs undertake a training on the treatment of water, they can go to a treatment plant to observe and learn from the actual processes. If a field site has a caretaker or individuals working there, it is important that they talk to the CHWs during the visit. Such field personnel normally have a wealth of knowledge on the subject that trainees would benefit from. Field visits normally ensure the CHWs appreciate the issues of concern, and this can facilitate use of the knowledge in the future. Indeed, observing procedures being conducted as part of the field trip is likely to leave memorable and lasting impressions among the trainees.

Before the field visit, CHWs can be taught about the subject of concern to get a general and theoretical understanding. In such an instance, the field trip would provide further in-depth comprehension on the topic of the training. Unlike other in-class training methods, field trips need logistical support such as transport, including a vehicle and fuel, which could be costly. In addition, some field sites could be very far away, with considerable cost implications. In certain circumstances, field sites may not grant permission for trainees to access them, which is another limitation of the method. Some local areas may also have no available field sites to be used for the training, thus limiting the use of the approach. Such logistical concerns therefore need to be considered during the planning of a training that involves field visits. Otherwise, other training approaches with fewer limitations, could be explored, as they may be more appropriate.

Gallery Walks

Gallery walks are an interactive mode of learning in which trainees move around different stations in small groups and explore a topic/question of interest in detail. This method, which can be used during training of CHWs, promotes critical thinking, cooperation, and knowledge sharing (Dinata, 2017). In the planning for a gallery walk, the facilitator needs to have several stations in the training room where interaction and discussions will take place. These stations should have the question or topic for discussion which could be on a computer, flip chart, or piece of paper. In small groups, CHWs move from one station to another, discussing respective topics in detail. Depending on the issue of discussion, CHWs can spend between 5 to 15 minutes at each station before moving to the next. During the small group discussions, the facilitator can move around and interact with the CHWs during the activity. Where there is more than one facilitator, each one could be based at a station so as to actively engage the CHWs whenever they join them. For the success of this method, it is important that all members of the group actively participate in the discussions, and this should be supported by the facilitator.

After all trainees have moved through all the stations, a wrap-up session, in which individuals from the different groups give feedback to the entire group, can be held. This feedback session can also be used by the facilitator to answer any questions that the CHWs may have. There are several benefits of using gallery walks in training CHWs, including improving communication skills, building teamwork, making learning interesting, reducing boredom from sitting in one place, and facilitating learning from experiences of the trainees (Ismail et al., 2017). It is important that the groups do not spend more time at each station than allocated, otherwise the entire session could take longer than planned. If the training involves many CHWs, the facility should have enough space for the gallery walks.

Class Presentations

Class presentations can be used during training of CHWs to enhance participation and foster learning. Such presentations can be employed after various training activities, such as group work, exercises, and field work. Making presentations by CHWs in front of colleagues builds their confidence, enhances communication skills, and facilitates collaborative learning (Thompson et al., 2012). Indeed, CHWs who have undertaken training involving presentations are likely to be more confident in talking to large groups of people during the course of their work. Given that many CHWs are involved in health promotion among communities as part of their roles, being able to communicate well is of paramount importance. Presentations can be made using PowerPoint slides, which would require certain logistics such as a projector and laptop. This may be unfavourable to CHWs with low levels of education. Preparing slides is another skill that CHWs can develop if they use them during training. Using audiovisuals during presentations makes the process interesting and prepares CHWs to potentially use them during their future work.

Making presentations also enables CHWs to provide feedback to each other, which enhances participatory learning and teamwork. The feedback provided by the facilitator after the presentations is important to offer guidance to the CHWs. In particular, the facilitator should be able to provide suggestions for improvement on presentation style, communication skills, and any other aspects geared towards making them better communicators. CHWs who may not have experience of standing in front of many people could find making presentations a daunting task. Nevertheless, the facilitator can support such individuals to ensure that they are able to learn this new skill. If several presentations are made during the course of a long-term training programme of CHWs, their skills in the activity are likely to improve, which would manifest in their enhanced confidence and communication. Presentations are therefore considered a key participatory training method that can be employed among CHWs.

Practicals

Practicals are a good training method for CHWs to give them hands-on exposure to a subject (Aitken, 2014). Such practicals provide CHWs with skills to use in the course of their work. Practicals can be used on a subject that requires CHWs to use a specialized skill during practice. Indeed, given the various roles of CHWs in promoting public health and primary healthcare in various settings, the ability to carry out some hands-on investigations in the community is of paramount importance. As an example, during training on water quality testing, practicals can be used so that CHWs have the knowledge and skills to carry out the tests. Such tests can include measurement of physical, chemical, and biological parameters in water, including pH and turbidity. Therefore, a practical session on use of pH and turbidity meters can be incorporated in a CHW training programme. Practicals for such tests are crucial if the CHWs are expected to use them during their work in communities. Otherwise, it is unlikely that CHWs would attempt to carry out such tests without having had any practical exposure.

It is important to note that some practicals require equipment which has to be available to the CHWs during training. As some equipment could be expensive, it may be unlikely that separate equipment is available for every CHW involved in the training. However, sharing equipment should ensure that every CHW gets enough exposure to enhance their skills for future practice. In addition, some practicals may require reagents and consumables such as gloves which could also be expensive in some settings. Access to electricity may also be needed to operate certain equipment that may not always be available, particularly in rural areas in LMICs. However, use of portable equipment, that can be operated using batteries of other forms of energy, such as solar, can be explored in such circumstances. Therefore, when considering practicals as a method for training CHWs, the availability and cost of equipment, as well as other requirements, need to be considered.

Case Studies

Case studies are real-life experiences that can be incorporated into training of CHWs as a means of learning from past occurrences. Such case studies can be helpful for scenarios in which previous events can enhance participants' understanding and learning (Davis & Wilcock, 2003). As case studies provide real-life examples (Raju & Sankar, 1999), including problems, solutions, and challenges, they make training sessions more interesting and memorable to trainees. The past event in a case study can be from the local setting of the trainees or other national or global locality. For example, a recent cholera outbreak in the community, or previous Ebola outbreak in West Africa, could be used as case studies while training CHWs on their role in outbreak investigation and control.

During the training, the case study can be read to the trainees, written on a board, or given to them for individual reading. The case study used should clearly bring out the event of concern, which should be emphasized by the facilitator. The facilitator can then use the occurrence to point out what was done well, what went wrong, and what could have been done better during the event. Otherwise, the facilitator may ask the trainees to mention the positives and negatives from the case study to stimulate discussion. In addition, the facilitator can ask the trainees to share their views on what they would have done if they were in a similar situation. Such questions to trainees enable them to reflect on the case study, and relate it to their own personal situation and experience. The particular lessons to be learnt from the event need to be emphasized to the CHWs for purposes of the training. In situations where a real-life case study cannot be found, a fictitious one can be used for the training. Case studies are useful in providing participants with realistic simulations of what they are likely to encounter during the course of their work. Some of the specific skills CHWs are likely to gain from engaging with case studies include problem identification, analysing information, critical thinking, making judgements, and taking decisions (International Council on Archives, 2005). Such skills are not only useful during the training but also in future day-to-day activities of CHWs in the community.

Interactive Exercises and Games

Interactive exercises and games can be used in training of CHWs to enhance learning, facilitate teamwork, and keep trainees interested and engaged. Various exercises and games can be used, such as icebreakers, energizers, and interactive games (Biech, 2008). Icebreakers are normally used as a fun activity for trainees and facilitators to get to know each other, as well as make participants feel relaxed (DeSilets, 2008). Such icebreakers can be used at the start of training to make CHWs more comfortable, and enhance their participation. Energizers can be used during the course of training as a form of interactive session to provide interludes in long activities (Chlup & Collins, 2010). Such energizers are helpful to enable the trainees take an interactive break, and ensure that they are ready for the next session. Besides icebreakers and energizers, other interactive games can be used during training of CHWs. These games can be organized based on specific topics of the training as a fun way to facilitate learning.

It should be noted that excessive use of interactive exercises can become monotonous and boring to trainees. In addition, having very many exercises may interrupt the flow of other aspects of the training. For a long-term training programme, it is important that new games are introduced to reduce monotony and keep trainees interested and motivated, which may be challenging to the facilitator. In some instances, trainees could be given the opportunity to introduce some of their own interactive games, which can be exciting to them. It is therefore important that interactive exercises and games are used judiciously to support the training objectives. During planning of interactive sessions, several issues should be considered such as physical space/setting of the venue, level of education of trainees, cultural differences of trainees, mobility of participants, and language.

Conclusion

Several methods to facilitate participatory training of CHWs have been presented, with the advantages and disadvantages of each summarized in Table 8.1. In choosing which training methods to use in CHW programmes, it is important to consider several factors, such as the number, level of education and experience of trainees; the resources available, including time, materials, and technology; as well as the topic and context of the training. The potential of technology, such as mobile technologies and the Internet, in supporting/enhancing learning is discussed in other chapters in this volume, and its feasibility should be considered as part of participatory training approaches. Participatory methods such as role-plays, group discussions and exercises are likely to be ideal in most settings. However, some methods, such as simulations, gallery walks, and field trips are more dependent upon space, planning, and resources and will be less feasible in some training sessions.

As much as is possible, methods chosen for use should ensure CHWs are at the centre of the training, with their full engagement in the learning process. There is evidence that active participation of CHWs in training not only makes it interesting to them but also enhances retention, confidence, and long-lasting change (Hill-Briggs et al., 2007). However, even when a certain method has previously been used elsewhere, it is always crucial to consider the local context while planning for its use in training CHWs. Despite the differences between the individual participatory training approaches, they all share the aim of empowering trainees by offering space to trainees and trainers not only for participation and action, but also for critical (self)-reflection. Together, reflection and action not only equalize the relationship between trainers and trainees and enhance the learning experience of CHWs, but ultimately lay the essential foundation for continuous learning and professional practice, so that these can inform the CHWs' daily work throughout their careers.

Table 8.1 Summary of participatory approaches for training CHWs

Method	Advantages	Disadvantages
Role-plays	• Can depict real-life scenarios • Useful for difficult or unfamiliar scenarios • Improve communication among trainees • Are enjoyable	• Could take a lot of time • Passive involvement of some trainees
Demonstrations	• Can provide a practical illustration of a task or technique • Enhance observational learning • Improve understanding of complex skills and techniques	• May not be suitable for large groups • Are time consuming
Songs	• Can be fun • Ideal for trainees with low education • Enhance creativity if songs are developed by trainees • Could be used by trainees during their own practice	• Require experienced facilitator
Small and large group discussions	• High level of learner involvement • Good utilization of learner knowledge and experiences	• Require a lot of time • Need to be adequately controlled
Brainstorming	• Explores learners' perspectives and experiences • Good to generate ideas • Good to understand the level of knowledge of trainees • Can be used as a precursor to other methods	• Requires adequate moderation • Time consuming • Some trainees could dominate
Debates	• Ideal for complex or controversial topics • Can be used for topics that could have divergent views • Can be used as a precursor before use of another method • Enhance capacity of trainees in public speaking • Stimulate thinking	• Could be challenging to learners with low education • Require experienced facilitator/moderator • Are time consuming
Simulations	• Can depict real-life scenarios • Useful for scenarios that are difficult to demonstrate • Provide hands-on experience • Can test proficiency in performing certain tasks	• Could be expensive • May not always be possible

(Continued)

Table 8.1 *Continued*

Method	Advantages	Disadvantages
Exercises	• High level of participation • Can take various forms such as written, oral, practical, or a combination • Can test mastery of a subject	• Could be demotivating if trainees fail • Are time consuming • May be challenging to provide individual feedback to all trainees
Field trips	• Enhance observing real-life activities • Active involvement of trainees	• Require much resources and logistics • Are normally time consuming • Need much planning • Dependent on external factors such as host institution
Gallery walks	• Promote critical thinking, cooperation, and knowledge sharing • Improve communication skills • Make learning interesting • Reduce boredom of sitting in one place	• Are time consuming • Require close facilitation • Require large training space • Need substantial amount of planning
Class presentations	• Enhance trainee participation • Build confidence • Enhance communication skills	• May require logistics such as a projector and laptop • May be time consuming
Practicals	• Give hands-on exposure	• Require much resources and logistics • May be time consuming
Case studies	• Can provide real-life examples • Interesting and memorable • Can stimulate discussion	• May not always be from the setting/context of interest
Interactive exercises and games	• Are fun • Enable trainees to know each other • Enhance bonding among trainees	• Could become monotonous and boring

References

Aggarwal, R., Mytton, O.T., Derbrew, M., Hananel, D., Heydenburg, M., Issenberg, B., et al. (2010). Training and simulation for patient safety. *BMJ Quality & Safety*, 19, i34–i43.

Aitken, I. (2014). Training community health workers for large-scale community-based health care programs. In: H. Perry & L. Crigler (Eds). *Developing and Strengthening Community Health Worker Programs at Scale: A Reference Guide and Case Studies for Program Managers and Policymakers*. Baltimore, Jhpiego, Chapter 9, pp. 9–24.

Basheer, A., Hugerat, M., Kortam, N., & Hofstein, A. (2017). The effectiveness of teachers' use of demonstrations for enhancing students' understanding of and attitudes to learning the oxidation-reduction concept. *Eurasia Journal of Mathematics, Science and Technology Education*, 13(3), 555–570. doi:10.12973/eurasia.2017.00632a.

Baum, F., MacDougall, C., & Smith, D. (2006). Participatory action research. *Journal of Epidemiology and Community Health*, 60(10), 854–857.

Biech, E. (Editor) (2008). *The Trainer's Warehouse Book of Games: Fun and Energizing Ways to Enhance Learning*. San Francisco, Pfeiffer.

CDC–Centers for Disease Control and Prevention (2009). *A Handbook for Enhancing CHW Programs: Guidance for the National Breast and Cervical Cancer Early Detection Program (Part 1)*. Available from: https://www.chwcentral.org/handbook-enhancing-community-health-worker-programs-guidance-national-breast-and-cervical-cancer

Chlup, D.T. & Collins, T.E. (2010). Breaking the ice: Using ice-breakers and Re-energizers with adult learners. *Adult Learning*, 21(3–4), 34–39.

Davis, C. & Wilcock, E. (2003). *Teaching Materials Using Case Studies. The UK Centre for Materials Education*. Available from: http://www.materials.ac.uk/guides/casestudies.asp

DeSilets, L. (2008). Using icebreakers to open communication. *Journal of Continuing Education in Nursing*, 39, 292–293.

Dinata, H. (2017). The use of gallery walk to enhance the speaking achievement of the ninth grade students of SMP PGRI 1 Palembang. *Global Expert Journal Bahasa Dan Sastra*, 6(1), 53–55.

Fournier-Sylvester, N. (2013). Daring to debate: Strategies for teaching controversial issues in the classroom. *College Quarterly*, 16(3), 1–9.

Freire, P. 1968. *Pedagogy of the Oppressed*. New York, Continuum.

Gogus, A. (2013). Brainstorming and invention. In: E.G. Carayannis (Ed.). *Encyclopedia of Creativity, Invention, Innovation and Entrepreneurship*. New York, Springer.

Healthy Child Uganda (2015). *Village Health Team Maternal Newborn and Child Health Training Manual*. Mbarara, Uganda.

Hill-Briggs, F., Batts-Turner, M., Gary, T.L., Brancati, F.L., Hill, M., Levine, D.M., et al. (2007). Training community health workers as diabetes educators for urban African Americans: Value added using participatory methods. *Progress in Community Health Partnerships: Research, Education, and Action*, 1(2), 185–194.

International Council on Archives. 2005. Developing and using case studies. Available from: http://www.ica-sae.org/trainer/english/p9.htm

Ismail, I., Sri Anitah, W., Sunardi, S., & Rochsantiningsih D. (2017). The effectiveness of gallery walk and simulation (GALSIM) to improve students' achievement in Fiqh learning. *Walisongo: Jurnal Penelitian Sosial Keagamaan*, 25(1), 231–252.

Kusnierek, A. (2016). The role of music and songs in teaching English vocabulary to students. *World Scientific News*, 43, 1–55.

Lateef, F. (2010). Simulation-based learning: Just like the real thing. *Journal of Emergencies, Trauma and Shock*, 3(4), 348–352. doi:10.4103/0974-2700.70743.

Ments, M.V. (1999). *The Effective Use of Role Play: Practical Techniques for Improving Learning* (Second Edition). London, Kogan Page.

Meo, S.A. (2013). Basic steps in establishing effective small group teaching sessions in medical schools. *Pakistan Journal of Medical Sciences*, 29(4), 1071–1076.

Millennium Villages Project (2013). *Community Health Worker Trainer's Manual. A Guide to Home-Based Services*. Millennium Villages Project at the Earth Institute of Colombia University.

Mohan, S.K. (2010). Participatory training methods. Available from: https://www.slideshare.net/subinkmohan/participatory-training-methods-by-dr-subin-mohan

Myers, B. & Jones, L. (2018). *Effective Use of Field Trips in Educational Programming: A Three Stage Approach*. University of Florida, UF/IFAS Extension, Agricultural Education and Communication Department. Available from: https://edis.ifas.ufl.edu/pdffiles/WC/WC05400.pdf

Naugle, D.A. & Hornik, R.C. (2014). Systematic review of the effectiveness of mass media interventions for child survival in low- and middle-income countries. *Journal of Health Communication*, 19(1), 190–215.

Pretty, J., Guijt, I., Thompson, J., & Scoones, I. (1995). *Participatory learning and action: A trainer's guide*. International Institute for Environment and Development Participatory Methodology Series, London.

PRIA–Society for Participatory Research in Asia (2013). *Participatory Learning and Training*. Available from: http://www.practiceinparticipation.org/index.php/pages/learning-and-training/

Raju, P.K. & Sankar, C.S. (1999). Teaching real-world issues through case studies. *Journal of Engineering Education*, 88(4), 501–509.

Rasul, S., Bukhsh, Q., & Batool, S. (2011). A study to analyze the effectiveness of audio visual aids in teaching learning process at university level. *Procedia—Social and Behavioral Sciences*, 28, 78–81.

Sfard, A. (1998). On two metaphors for learning and the dangers of choosing just one. *Educational Researcher*, 27(2), 4–13.

Smartsheet (2019). *Discover the Best Brainstorming Approaches and Techniques to Motivate Your Team*. Available from: https://www.smartsheet.com/brainstorming-techniques-activities-and-exercises

Špernjak, A. & Šorgo, A. (2018). Differences in acquired knowledge and attitudes achieved with traditional, computer-supported and virtual laboratory biology laboratory exercises. *Journal of Biological Education*, 52(2), 206–220.

Stokoe, E. (2011). Simulated interaction and communication skills training: The 'conversation-analytic role-play method'. In: C. Antaki (Ed.). *Applied Conversation Analysis. Palgrave Advances in Linguistics*. London, Palgrave Macmillan.

Thompson, K.J., Switky, B., & Gilinsky, A. (2012). Impromptu presentations: Boosting student learning and engagement through spontaneous collaboration. *Journal of Education for Business*, 87(1), 14–21.

Van Boetzelaer, E., Zhou, A., Tesfai, C., & Kozuki, N. (2019). Performance of low-literate community health workers treating severe acute malnutrition in South Sudan. *Maternal & Child Nutrition*, 15(1), e12716.

World Health Organization (2018). *WHO Guideline on Health Policy and System Support to Optimize Community Health Worker Programmes*. Geneva, World Health Organization. Licence: CC BY-NC-SA 3.0 IGO.

Wikipedia. 2019. Debates. Available from: https://en.wikipedia.org/wiki/Debate

9

The Danger of a Single Study

Developing Responsive Evidence Bases to Inform Research, Policy, and Practice on the Training of Community Health Workers in Low and Middle-Income Countries

Promise Nduku, Nkululeko Tshabalala, Moshidi Putuka, Zafeer Ravat, and Laurenz Langer

Introduction

The danger of a single story is not that they are untrue but that they are incomplete. This is the key message from Chimamanda Ngozi Adichie seminal Ted Talk (Adichie, 2016) in which she outlines the risks of one dominant view crowding out different perspectives. The same concept applies to single research studies. It is not that single studies are flawed or incorrect; to the contrary, the vast majority of single studies are highly accurate and trustworthy in their findings. However, in the context of decision-making for policy and practice, single studies—just as single stories—should not become the only story for decision makers. For effective and equitable decision-making, we need to hear all the stories; and hence, we need to access all the studies in order to compile an evidence base that can mitigate against the danger of a single study.

The negative consequences of using single studies to inform decision-making have been well established in a range of sectors, including education and health. From the myth of learning styles to virtual infant parenting programmes (Stewart et al., 2018), single studies, discourses, and paradigms have often skewed decision-making to ineffective and sometimes harmful interventions. The same trend can be observed in the context of training community health workers (CHWs) in low and middle-income countries (LMICs). For example, single trials of individual CHWs programmes are taken as proof of effectiveness and used to justify large-scale funding investments (c.f. Winters et al., 2019).

With increased interest and subsequent research production on identifying the most effective and relevant models to train CHWs, it seems an opportune moment to argue, first, for a shift of focus in research production away from single studies and towards systematic evidence bases and synthesis of CHW-focused research, and, second, for a similar shift in what types of research evidence decision makers are using

Promise Nduku, Nkululeko Tshabalala, Moshidi Putuka, Zafeer Ravat, and Laurenz Langer, *The Danger of a Single Study*
In: *Training for Community Health*. Edited by: Anne Geniets, James O'Donovan, Laura Hakimi, and Niall Winters,
Oxford University Press. © Oxford University Press 2021. DOI: 10.1093/oso/9780198866244.003.0009

to inform the design and implementation of CHWs training programmes. In this chapter, we develop this argument and outline, based on our experience of working with policymakers in South Africa, an approach to compile responsive evidence bases to inform research, policy, and practice on the training of CHWs in LMICs.

The chapter is structured as follows: we first discuss the role of knowledge translation and evidence-informed decision-making (EIDM) to support the practice of CHWs and their training. This is followed by an outline of the specific contribution that evidence synthesis can make to support EIDM for CHWs. Next, we introduce different types of evidence synthesis before zooming in on one specific type—evidence maps—in the fourth section of the chapter. We conclude with a brief discussion.

Knowledge Translation and Evidence-Informed Practice for the Training of CHWs in LMICs

CHWs fulfil a critical function in supporting the provision of essential health services in LMICs. There is strong evidence of CHWs' positive contribution to delivering basic and essential health services and improving health outcomes such as reproductive and maternal health (e.g. Gilmore et al., 2013), infectious and non-communicable diseases (e.g. van Ginneken et al., 2013; Mwai et al., 2013) and neglected tropical diseases (e.g. Vouking et al., 2013). However, despite their proven potential to support health systems, CHWs are often not fully integrated and recognized for their contribution (WHO, 2018). This is particularly acute in the context of the training of CHWs, which often overlooks the individual learning and empowerment of CHWs as health practitioners in favour of training approaches that are task- and process-focused, leaving little room for the growth and development of CHWs (Winters et al., 2019).

The Current State of Evidence-Informed Practice and CHWs

The training and education of CHWs is also one of the key areas in which evidence-based practice guidelines are still underdeveloped or lacking altogether (WHO, 2018). For example, the WHO is unable to recommend specific education approaches or supervision strategies for CHW due to an evidence base that is described as 'not sufficiently granular' (WHO, 2018, p. 17). This lack of evidence-based educational practice guidelines presents a major barrier to the effective and equitable training of CHWs and subsequent personal empowerment and contribution to health systems. This chapter will adopt Langer and colleagues; (2016, p. 6) definition of evidence-based practice[1] as: 'a process whereby multiple sources of information, including the

---

[1] From here on we will prefer the term evidence-informed over evidence-based to indicate that evidence presents but one factor in the decision-making process (for a more detailed discussion, see Stewart et al., 2017).

best available research evidence, are consulted before making a decision to plan, implement, and (where relevant) alter policies, programmes and other services'.

The Benefits of Using Evidence

The training of CHWs in LMICs can gain from taking an evidence-informed approach in three ways. First, designing training programmes on the basis of 'theories unsupported by reliable empirical evidence' is irresponsible–and arguably unethical —as it leaves as much potential to do harm as to do good (Chalmers, 2005, p. 229). Exposing CHWs to training approaches based on educational theories and practices untested for their relevance to the contexts in which CHWs operate, can be regarded as akin to experimenting on CHWs. Educational approaches and principles, in particular where they are transferred from the Global North to the Global South, need to be carefully reviewed, based on the existing evidence base for their relevance, effectiveness, and equity implications in the contexts in which CHWs in LMICs operate.

Second, using evidence systematically can separate effective training programmes from ineffective ones and avoid wasting funds on the latter. This economic rationale for EIDM applies in LMICs in particular. LMICs have fewer resources at their disposal to fund health services and low-income groups in these countries are most dependent on the provision of public services. Every training programme that does not achieve its objective of supporting CHWs to deliver enhanced and improved health services, carries a large opportunity cost and missed developmental objective. By one estimate, as much as 85% of health research—to a total value of $200 billion in 2010 alone—is wasted by not being accessible and usable by health policymakers and practitioners (Chalmers & Glasziou, 2009).

Third, from an equity perspective, the integration of a diverse body of research evidence in the decision-making process opens this process to a wider range of perspectives. A range of structural inequalities—along lines of sex, location, education, to name a few—have historically affected access to decision-making processes. Research evidence representing different populations, voices, and perspectives, can provide an entry point and vehicle for groups and ideas with less access to decision makers. In the case of women's empowerment and representation, for example, data on inequalities based on sex first entered decision-making processes before the actual women themselves did (Oakley, 2000). This is particularly relevant to the issue of CHW recognition and empowerment. Many training programmes for CHWs are not based on evidence that has been at least co-produced by CHWs themselves. A systematic practice of using a diverse range of evidence, especially evidence from CHWs themselves, presents a large opportunity to design more effective and equitable programmes.

In summary, there is a strong moral imperative to support the use of evidence to inform the training of CHWs in LMICs. Research evidence can play an important role in designing and implementing training programmes for CHWs. And, this is by no means a theoretical discussion. In South Africa, effective knowledge translation on

HIV/AIDS policy and programming, including a more evidence-informed approach to the integration of CHWs, has been estimated to have prevented a total of 1.72 million deaths in the country between 2000–2014 (Suthar et al., 2017).

From Single Studies to Responsive Evidence Bases

So far, we have outlined the overall need for EIDM and have introduced the danger of the single study. This then leaves the question of what evidence should be used to inform decisions-making for the training of CHWs? We would suggest *responsive evidence bases* to be the most relevant source of evidence to support EIDM for CHWs.

Evidence Bases for Decision-Making

Over the last decade, the body of evidence on CHWs in LMICs has grown rapidly (WHO, 2018; Winters et al., 2019). However, this rapid growth of research is largely clustered in primary studies rather than syntheses of research (WHO, 2018). That is, there is a relative lack of evidence synthesis and other research products that compile a body of existing primary studies. This pattern risks that decisions on what types of training programmes to implement are often based on single evaluations of programmes conducted elsewhere; and that programme design considerations are informed by generic educational principles rather than contextualized learning strategies. There are a number of examples of the outsized influence of single studies, in particular programme evaluations and trials, on decision-making and programme funding such as the case of the randomized controlled trial (RCT) of the Living Goods programme (Nyqvist et al., 2019; Winters et al., 2019).

Targeting evidence bases, rather than single studies, also reinforces each of the moral imperatives for EIDM introduced in section 1.2. An assessment of the potential harms and benefits of a training programme is more reliable if it is based on a number of evaluations conducted across contexts than if it is based on a single evaluation. Likewise, the larger the body of available evidence, the more diverse the perspectives and voices that this evidence base can represent for consideration during decision-making. In addition to merely reinforcing directions and reliability of findings, oftentimes new meta-patterns can only be identified in the totality of evidence. The logo of the Cochrane Collaboration, for example, represents the results of a seminal meta-analysis, which overturned prevailing non-administration of corticosteroids to women who are about to give birth prematurely (Cochrane, 2020). The combined results of the existing trials revealed a strong pattern of effectiveness for the intervention that an observation of the single studies in isolation would have not identified.

Furthermore, evidence bases provide a more comprehensive assessment of the interplay of intervention implementation and contextual factors in complex social settings and how any research results can be transferred across such contexts. The training of CHWs is a social intervention, not a medical intervention. The complexities of transferring the results of intervention implementation in one social setting to another are vast and multiple once the differences in the training design itself are factored in too. In order to assess the likelihood of intervention results being transferable across different contexts, we require data on the different contexts in which CHWs operate, how these contexts interplay with different training designs, and what mechanisms drive intervention effects.

Given the rise in primary studies on the training of CHWs, this information is available at the individual study level. However, as noted in the WHO guidelines on CHWs, good practice and evidence-based design features for CHWs programmes are not replicated across contexts and there is little uniformity in policies across health ministries in LMICs (WHO, 2018). This is a missed opportunity for learning from the accumulated and combined evidence base on training of CHWs. Without tapping into this evidence base, the transferability and external validity of individual CHWs training programmes will remain challenged.

Last, there is also a strong pragmatic case for the advocacy of using evidence bases for decision-making. In the Information Age, such syntheses of bodies of evidence have become ever-more demanded by health and education policymakers and practitioners (Mijumbi et al., 2017; Stewart et al., 2019). Given the challenging task to keep up with the increasing rate of research publication, big data, and short time frames in which decisions have to be made, decision makers simply do not have the time and resources to access and make sense of all the individual primary studies. Systematically collated and appraised evidence bases greatly reduce the need to search for evidence, assess its trustworthiness and relevance, and aggregate and configure the overall research results. Consequently, evidence syntheses are a good fit for the rapid time frame and complex evidence needs of CHWs policymakers and programme designers.

Responsiveness as a Key Attribute of the Evidence Base

Enhancing the supply of evidence bases alone, however, is unlikely to systematically improve the use of evidence to inform the design of training programmes for CHWs (Parkhurst, 2017). We similarly need to support the demand for evidence by CHW decision makers. A key mechanism in this effort is to better match the available evidence base to research, policy, and practice needs. This can be achieved by enhancing the 'responsiveness' of these evidence bases. Responsiveness in this context refers to evidence bases that are: (1) produced in a time frame that matches decision making processes; (2) relevant to and driven by decision-makers' evidence needs; (3) accessible and usable by decision makers without researcher involvement; and (4) perceived as trustworthy and legitimate by decision makers.

In order to meet the above requirement of responsiveness, bodies of evidence need to consist of as broad as possible types of research studies. No single type of studies, for example RCTs or ethnographies, can address all decision-making needs.

And, decision makers need access to not just formal research studies but, equally important, practitioner and patient feedback, policy documents, implementation and project reports, data sources (e.g. census data), and more. This body of information, often referred to as grey literature, is critical in compiling an evidence base that is tailored according to decision-making priorities.

Given this broad evidence base, CHW decision makers need to be empowered to recognize the trade-offs between different types of evidence and the specific demands on evidence in policy and practice contexts. While the rigour or trustworthiness of the evidence is important, its relevance to the specific decision-making context, and its legitimacy in the eyes of the policy and practice stakeholders are equally important attributes to consider. For example, decision makers might prioritize local and more context-relevant evidence over more rigorous evidence conducted in less relevant contexts.

The accessibility of the evidence base is a further key criterion for its responsiveness. Systematic reviews and other types of evidence synthesis are usually presented in the form of long technical reports with a shorter summary and/or policy brief. Such static outputs are unlikely to meet rapidly changing decision-making needs and contexts. Responsive evidence bases therefore need to be directly accessible by decision makers and enable them to access the available evidence themselves and to tailor it to their contexts. This ability is provided by a range of IT applications, including evidence mapping tools (Snilstveit et al., 2016; Dayal & Langer, 2016), evidence portals (Gough & White, 2018), and interactive decision-making toolkits (Weyrauch, 2016).

Last, to produce responsiveness evidence bases, CHW decision makers require a much larger role in shaping the research process itself. Such involvement can range from a spectrum of stakeholder engagement (e.g. Haddaway & Crowe, 2017), priority setting and rapid feedback (e.g. Mijumbi et al., 2017), and full co-production (e.g. Dayal, 2019). Regardless of the format chosen, the involvement of decision makers serves to align and match the research process with policy and practice evidence needs. It ensures the developed evidence base is relevant and perceived as a legitimate input in the decision-making process. Having been directly involved in its production, decision makers have more ownership and control over the body of evidence, which supports its integration in often highly political decision-making processes.

Methodologies to Develop Responsive Evidence Bases

There are a range of different methodologies to develop responsive evidence bases. The common core of these methodologies is to collect a body of evidence in a systematic and transparent manner and to then synthesize the results of the collected individual studies. This process of *evidence synthesis* aims to understand the totality of evidence and to develop a body of knowledge that is more than the sum of its parts. This science of evidence synthesis is most commonly associated with the methodology of systematic reviews (Gough et al., 2017), which were first produced at scale in the healthcare sector following the foundation of the Cochrane Foundation in 1993.

Systematic reviews have since been established in a range of fields outside health, including education, international development, environmental science, and more (Langer & Stewart, 2014). Systematic review methods as the gold standard for evidence synthesis have evolved further too, often in response to policy and practitioners' needs for relevant and trustworthy evidence. This had led to a broader range of methodologies under the method family of evidence synthesis, which are introduced briefly next.

Systematic Reviews

Systematic review is a research methodology to systematically and transparently identify, access, appraise, and synthesize all available research studies on a given research question or topic. Formally, systematic review can be defined as: 'a review of research literature using systematic and explicit, accountable methods' (Gough et al., 2017). The methodology's guiding principles are to be transparent and systematic at any step of the research process (Petticrew & Roberts, 2006; Oliver, 2014; Stewart, 2014). This translates into a set of methodological characteristics associated with any systematic review: a clearly stated set of objectives with pre-defined eligibility criteria for inclusion of primary studies; an explicit, reproducible methodology; a systematic search that attempts to identify all studies that would meet the eligibility criteria; an assessment of the validity of the findings of the included studies; a systematic presentation and synthesis of the characteristics and findings of the included studies (Higgins et al., 2011; Gough et al., 2017; Stewart, 2014).

There are different types of systematic reviews. While historically in the healthcare sector most reviews aimed to assess the effectiveness of medical interventions using statistical techniques to synthesize the reported effects of existing trials, reviews now cover the full spectrum of research and practice questions. This includes qualitative evidence synthesis (QES) to assess facilitators and barriers (Greenhalgh et al., 2005), conceptual syntheses to understand meta-theories (e.g. Dixon-Woods et al., 2005), reviews following realist principles (e.g. Pawson, 2006), to name a few. These diverse reviews have covered different questions related to CHWs, for example investigating the implementation of CHWs programmes (Glenton et al., 2013) and substantiating CHWs' positive effect on a range of healthcare practices such as immunization uptake (Lewin et al., 2010).

Rapid Reviews

Rapid review presents a method that has been tailored to conduct an evidence synthesis in a more timely and relevant fashion without compromising the key principles of systemic reviews—transparency, and following a structured and reproducible process. In the context of healthcare interventions, rapid reviews have been defined as 'a type of knowledge synthesis in which systematic review processes are accelerated and methods are streamlined to complete the review more quickly than is the case for typical systematic reviews' (Tricco et al., 2017, p. 3). Outside healthcare, rapid review types have been conducted under different labels, such as rapid evidence assessment, rapid technology assessment, responsive evidence synthesis (Van Rooyen et al., forthcoming). Across disciplines, a rapid review is expected not to take longer than three months, while the average systematic review is produced between 12 to 24 months (Tricco et al., 2017).

Rapid reviews have emerged out of the need to conduct systematic evidence synthesis in a more timely and relevant fashion. Users of systematic reviews, in particular policymakers, have long cited reviews' time frame, cost, and lack of user engagement as key barriers for the application of reviews to decision-making (Oliver et al., 2016). In response, innovation in synthesis research, such as technology-assisted screening and embedded engagement, has led to a range of approaches to conduct 'quick and clean' evidence syntheses that meets users' needs on time and without compromising the rigour and transparency of more traditional reviews. The Centre for Rapid Evidence Synthesis at Makerere University in Uganda, in particular, has led this synthesis innovation and is providing a service for rapid evidence synthesis for the Ugandan Government that produces reviews within 3, 10, and 30 days (Mijumbi et al., 2017; Mijumbi & Sewankambo, 2018).

Evidence Maps

Evidence maps, alternatively called evidence gap maps or systematic maps, are a more recent addition to the family of evidence synthesis methods. Pioneered by the International Initiative for Impact Evaluation (3ie) (Snilstveit et al., 2013; 2016), they are now conducted by a number of organizations, including all systematic review umbrella organizations. As a methodology, evidence mapping systematically sources and organizes a body of knowledge to provide a high-level overview of the size and nature of the available evidence in order to inform and facilitate the use of this evidence base. That is, evidence maps are particularly concerned with the representation and accessibility of the overall body of evidence. Unlike systematic reviews, they therefore do not aim to provide answers to specific research and policy questions but target broad questions and the underlying characteristics and usability of the evidence base. In this, evidence maps commonly map the available body of knowledge against a schematic framework, for example an intervention-outcome framework or mechanism-context framework. Figure 9.1 below provides the schematic framework for an evidence map of CHW and education.

Evidence maps are particularly concerned with establishing two characteristics of the available body of evidence: the size and nature of the evidence. In terms of size, evidence maps indicate for which parts of the evidence base there is existing research available to inform decision makers; and, conversely, where there are research gaps in which insufficient evidence is available. In terms of nature, evidence maps then unpack the patterns within the existing evidence base. For example, this can include regional patterns in evidence production, what types of research studies have been conducted, and whether they are trustworthy, or what populations studies have focused on and if the available studies are sensitive to equity objectives (Kraemer-Mbula & Nduku, 2019).

In order to enhance usability, evidence maps provide an interactive mapping tool to visualize the evidence base and allow users to directly engage with the evidence base. For an example of such visualization interfaces see an evidence gap map[2] and evidence map[3]. Users can filter and contextualize the map according to their needs. They can also access the mapped evidence either as a structured summary or as a full text where studies are open access.

Other Types of Evidence Bases

Outside these three main approaches to developing responsive evidence bases, a number of related research methods are often mentioned. These include literature reviews, knowledge repositories/databases, meta-reviews, and practice guidelines. Each of these, however, has important drawbacks that hinder their classification as methods for developing responsive evidence bases. A detailed discussion of these is provided by Dayal and Langer (2016).

An Introduction to Developing Policy- and Practice-Relevant Evidence Bases to Guide the Training of CHWs in LMICs

Having briefly outlined the main methodologies for developing responsive evidence bases, we will now zoom in on evidence mapping to support policy- and practice-relevant evidence bases to guide the training of CHWs in LMICs. Of the range of evidence synthesis tools, we would posit evidence mapping as the most relevant method in the context of the training of CHWs. This assessment is based on three

---

[2] https://gapmaps.3ieimpact.org/evidence-maps/effect-transparency-and-accountability-interventions-extractive-sectors-evidence-gap
[3] https://africacentreforevidence.org/wp-content/uploads/2019/11/VAWC_v5-final_different-colours.html

observations: first, while not extensive in comparison to the available primary studies, a number of systematic reviews on the training of CHWs has been conducted. This includes reviews that answer questions of what training programmes works (e.g. O'Donovan et al., 2018) as well as why and how these programmes work (e.g. Glenton et al., 2013). However, such reviews are by definition focused on well-defined narrow questions of programme effectiveness and implementation.

Second, only a small number of rapid reviews of topics related to CHWs exist; and based on a search of academic databases none of these rapid reviews focus on the training of CHWs in LMICs. Based on the lessons learned of the only institution-alized rapid review service in Africa that spans the health and educations sectors, a major impediment to the conduct of rapid reviews is the unavailability of a pre-organized evidence base (Mijumbi et al., 2017; 2018). The time invested in searching for and screening relevant research studies is a major barrier to rapid evidence syn-thesis. Evidence maps in this context can present the repository and database used as a source to conduct rapid reviews. This model has been successfully institutionalized in the social sectors, including education by the South African Government (DPME, 2016; Dayal & Langer, 2019), who in 2020 have extended their rapid evidence re-sponse service to the health sector (DPME, 2020).

Third, for bodies of evidence to be useful and used for practice and policy decision-making, they need to be fully accessible by decision makers and tailor-made to their contexts. Evidence maps are the only evidence synthesis tool that pro-vides direct access to all the underlying primary evidence in one platform. Further, the interactive features of the mapping platform allow different policy and practice audiences to zoom in on and customize the evidence base relevant to their own needs. Maps thereby fill a large gap in the evidence ecosystem for the training of CHWs in LMICs, bridging the production, brokering, and use of evidence for deci-sion making.

Seven Steps to Developing Policy- and Practice-Relevant Evidence Bases

Evidence maps aim to provide a policy- and practice-relevant evidence base. This sets them apart from traditional systematic reviews and other types of evidence synthesis. To achieve this aim, maps adapt each step in the systematic review process and place a much stronger emphasis on user engagement. In our model for policy-relevant evidence maps in South Africa (Dayal & Langer, 2016), co-production between government and the research sector is embedded within the process of evidence mapping. While not all mapping approaches go as far as to advocate for embedded co-production, a synthesis of the different methods for evidence mapping confirms the centrality of deep user engagement in the production of maps (Miake-Lye et al., 2016). The adapted research steps in policy- and practice-relevant evidence maps are outlined in Table 9.1:

Table 9.1 Research steps in policy-relevant evidence maps

Step in the mapping process	Description
1 Develop a policy or practice narrative	A policy or practice narrative refers to a road map on how the map can be used for decision-making. Its development is led by the prospective users of the map and often based on existing policy and practice frameworks (e.g. white papers, practice guidelines). The narrative is the key tool to ensure the relevance and legitimacy of the produced evidence base. The output of the narrative directly informs the schematic mapping framework and defines the users' evidence needs.
2 Decide what constitutes relevant evidence	Relevant evidence refers to the type of research, information, and documentation that is regarded to be fit for purpose to inform decision-making. This is translated into explicit and transparent inclusion criteria. The emphasis is to develop criteria that are driven by users' evidence needs and thus often include broader criteria than in systematic reviews, with a strong emphasis on the inclusion of grey literature.
3 Search for evidence	A systematic and exhaustive search for evidence is conducted to ensure that no relevant evidence is missed for the map. This follows guidelines for scientific search strategies and is complemented by a detailed grey literature search to identify practice and policy knowledge.
4 Extract, categorize, and code data from evidence	The process of data extraction records all information from the included evidence that is relevant to inform decision-making. The emphasis in data extraction is to organize information to develop an evidence base that is responsive to practice and policy needs. Therefore, extraction focuses on data relevant for long-term evidence needs rather than once-off synthesis.
5 Appraise evidence	A critical appraisal is conducted to give decision makers an indication of the trustworthiness and relevance of the available evidence. This step combines a traditional assessment of the methodological rigour of studies (trustworthiness) with their relevance to policy and practice needs as well as their legitimacy to these audiences.
6 Present and visualize the evidence base	The evidence map is visualized on an interactive and user-friendly IT platform tailored to decision makers' needs and contexts (see Figure 9.1).
7 Engage and use evidence for decision-making	The main aim of the evidence map is to inform decision-making (see application in 'How Can Evidence Maps Inform Decision-Making Related to the Training of CHWs?'). This step relies heavily on the developed policy narrative and continued user engagement. The map aims to present a long-term evidence base that is responsive to changing evidence needs.

Step 6 in the mapping process deserves further illustration. As indicated above, most maps organize the included evidence in a schematic framework. This framework usually presents two variables, for example interventions and outcomes. In order to engage with the mapped evidence directly, an interactive evidence mapping tool is programmed. There are different software options available, which all follow the same concept outlined below using the example of the Africa Centre for Evidence's open-access software. The screenshots below used to illustrate the mapping tool's functionality that are based on an evidence map on the use of mobile technologies to support the training of CHWs in LMICs (Winters et al., 2019). The map works online and offline and can be accessed here: https://africacentreforevidence.org/project-outputs-6/

In Figure 9.1, the mapping framework is represented by the light gray top and left axes representing the underlying educational approach (left axis) and the health condition targeted (top axis) respectively. The size of the dark gray indicates the size of the available evidence: the larger the bubble, the larger the evidence base. The colour of the bubble can be further tailored to represent different attributes of the evidence base, for example the trustworthiness and relevance of the evidence or the degree to which the evidence base is focused on equity objectives (Kraemer-Mbula & Nduku, 2019).

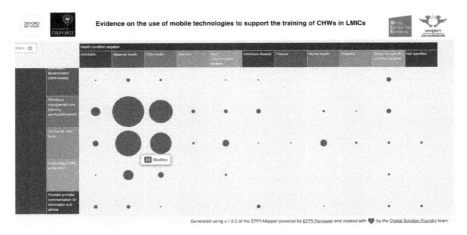

Figure 9.1 Example of an interactive evidence map.
Source: data from https://africacentreforevidence.org/project-outputs-6/

By clicking on a bubble, users can access the primary studies contained in it. A new pop up then opens indicating all individual studies and the meta-data associated with each (Figure 9.2). This interface also includes a URL to either the full text of the included study (if the study is open access) or to a structured summary of the study.

In addition, users can apply the filtering function (Figure 9.3) to tailor the evidence map according to their needs. This function allows users to filter the map by predefined variables such as region and study design, which then updates the evidence map to only show the evidence according to the user's specification. The filtering variables are chosen by users themselves in the policy narrative and data extraction stage.

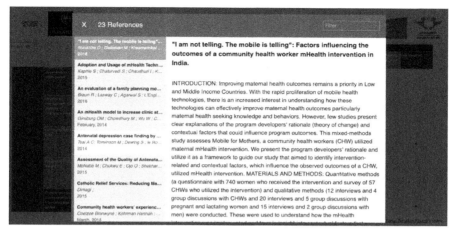

Figure 9.2 Accessing primary studies through the interactive evidence map.
Source: data from https://africacentreforevidence.org/project-outputs-6/

How Can Evidence Maps Inform Decision-Making Related to the Training of CHWs?

Evidence maps are a deliberate methodological attempt to make bodies of research more likely to be used by decision makers. They contribute a responsive evidence base to serve as a versatile tool to be applied by decision makers in policy and practice contexts. 'Responsive' here refers to the range of attributes of the developed evidence base outlined above. Evidence maps are directly integrated with the expressed

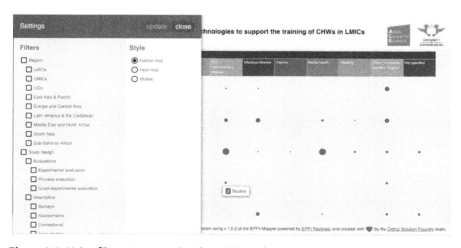

Figure 9.3 Using filters to customise the evidence base.
Source: data from https://africacentreforevidence.org/project-outputs-6/

evidence needs of decision makers (relevance); aligned with decision makers' time-lines and supporting rapid application (timeliness); produced with decision makers through extensive consultation (legitimacy); permanently accessible by decision makers in a user-friendly manner (accessibility); and produced to standard systematic review research processes and protocol (trustworthiness). In each of these, one needs to keep in mind that the maps present different bodies of evidence (e.g. in different bubbles) and thereby strongly encourage the use of evidence syntheses rather than single studies.

To further explore the relevance and application of evidence maps for decision makers, we gathered detailed feedback and input from South African policymakers at the Department of Planning, Monitoring, and Evaluation (DPME) involved in five evidence maps between 2016 and 2019. Based on these reflections and feedback, we identified ten applications of evidence maps in the process of using evidence to inform policymaking (Dayal & Langer, 2016). Evidence maps application as:

1. A *decision-making tool* to inform policy and practice. In specific contexts, evidence maps can be used to directly inform decision-making. For example, when the map indicates an absolute gap of evidence against a considered policy or practice option, this could support a decision to reconsider this option.

2. A *scoping tool* to inform a policy or practice theory of change and evaluation. More commonly, maps can be used in an instrumental sense to support the unpacking of a policy or programme. In particular, they can support the development of a theory of change for the policy or programme and safeguard that different building blocks of this theory of change are evidence informed. This supports the targeted evaluation of policies and programmes along a reliable theory of change.

3. A *validation tool* to comply with evidence standards and requirements. In contexts where decision makers work in organizations which have developed detailed evidence standards or requirements (e.g. NICE in the UK and SEIAS in South Africa) that need to be met for decision making, evidence maps can be used as the source database from which to draw this evidence to meet the required standards.

4. A *sourcing tool* for rapid response services. Evidence maps have shown strong synergies with rapid response services and other instruments for rapid syntheses of evidence. In situations where decision makers require rapid policy or practice answers (often within days), maps can be used as a primary source of evidence for this research service.

5. An *engagement tool* to facilitate conversations with different decision-making actors from a mutual basis. Evidence maps can be used to support engagement between different stakeholders in a decision-making process. Policy- and practice-relevant evidence maps cover a spectrum of evidence, including the current types of evidence that decision makers are already using. By

deliberately including this wide spectrum of evidence, they acknowledge the different existing evidence bases of stakeholders. This assures all parties that their respective evidence is considered and supports a decision-making dialogue departing from a mutual basis of recognition and trust.

6. A *knowledge management tool* providing a repository of easily accessible and relevant evidence tailored to decision-makers' needs. Evidence maps can be used to facilitate knowledge management and translation in policy and practice organizations. Maps constitute a knowledge repository but extend beyond this function of merely gathering and collecting evidence; they further organize and visualize the evidence base according to decision makers' priorities who can customize the maps to their own needs.

7. An *organizational tool* to raise awareness for EIDM and to facilitate its process. Evidence maps can be used to support an organization towards mainstreaming EIDM. They can be applied as an easy-to-use interactive tool to introduce decision makers to the idea of using evidence and to highlight that using evidence need not be a highly technical process.

8. An *accountability tool* to record the evidence behind a decision. Evidence maps can be used to support transparency in the decision-making process. Decision makers can illustrate that they have considered a wide body of evidence to inform their decisions. This can increase accountability in how a policy or practice decision has been reached and, likewise, set the scene for future evidence needs.

9. A *research tool* to identify gaps, coverage, and patterns in the available evidence base. Evidence maps can be used to understand the patterns in an existing evidence base and to juxtapose this evidence base with decision-making needs. They illustrate for which policy or practice priorities there is existing evidence and for which there is a lack of evidence. This can support organizations in formulating their own evidence needs and to develop a research and evidence strategy based on the current patterns in the evidence base.

10. A *research commissioning tool* to target funding for new primary and secondary evidence. Evidence maps can be used to support the commissioning of research evidence against the identified evidence gaps. This can either refer to gaps in the existing primary research or to gaps in the production of synthesis studies where there is sufficient primary evidence.

In sum, the above presents a range of possible application of evidence maps to support decision-making. While not directly based on experiences in the healthcare sector, the presented applications apply across sectors. The five evidence maps produced by DPME include the education, housing, urban planning, land reform, and public administration sector, with an evidence map on universal health insurance being produced. Policymakers, practitioners, and researchers concerned with the training of CHWs in the LMICs stand to benefit from applying evidence mapping more systematically to guide decision-making.

Discussion

Decision makers and researchers face many questions when identifying relevant approaches for the training of CHWs in LMICs. Effective training approaches will differ according to contexts, implementation considerations vary, and research is often subject to structural biases. Nevertheless, decision makers have little choice but to implement programmes even in the absence of full knowledge and presence of tight time frames and budgets. Having convenient access to a responsive evidence base that contains and organizes the relevant research and data on the training of CHWs in LMICs is but one type of support busy practitioners and policymakers should receive.

Based on our work in the South African policy sector, we have observed first-hand how responsive evidence bases can support decision-making. In the education sector, an evidence map was commissioned to inform the design of an multi-arm RCT helping to identify which interventions to include in the arms of the trial; in the housing sector, an evidence map was directly integrated into the white paper policy development process to support stakeholder engagement to build a joint foundation on which to discuss conflicting policy stances; and in the land reform sector, an evidence map was produced to support a rapid three-day synthesis to triangulate the evidence base behind different policy recommendations (Dayal, 2019; Langer, 2019).

These examples have direct relevance to decision-making concerning the training of CHWs in LMICs. Based just on the single evidence map on the use of mobile technologies to support the training of CHWs in LMICs, we can see which areas would most benefit from the commissioning of new research and which areas of research are rather saturated (Winters et al., 2019). We can also see structural patterns in the evidence base: in which countries is research clustered; who conducts research on CHWs in LMICs—researchers based in the Global North or South; and which research approaches dominate.

As in the case of the housing sector in South Africa, we require a mutual basis for discussion on the training and CHWs sector too. Many conversations on the training of CHWs take place in silos. These can be sectoral silos (e.g. health vs. education), discipline silos (workplace based learning vs. formal learning) or regional silos, to name a few. Starting conversations on a shared foundation of evidence has the potential to make these conversations more meaningful and to accelerate cross-learning and the creation of synergies. And, as in the case of land reform in South Africa, by developing responsive evidence bases, we can rapidly, within days, understand what works, why, and how. This ability is especially relevant in health emergencies such as Ebola or the coronavirus outbreak. Finally, we can move towards the institutionalization of the embedding of evidence bases in decision-making, which has been pioneered in the health sector by ACRES at Makerere University. Such African evidence innovations can inspire a sustained evidence-informed practice in the training of CHWs in LMICs.

By no means does any of this suggest that evidence maps or any form of evidence synthesis is an end in itself or silver bullet to support EIDM. Various studies have investigated the many mechanisms to support the use of research evidence (e.g. Nutley et al., 2007; Langer et al., 2016). A common finding across these investigations is that: (1) trusted interactions between evidence producers and users; (2) skills and motivation of evidence users; and (3) institutional support structures and processes are key to the practice of using evidence. These findings seem to be particularly relevant in the context of empowering CHWs themselves to engage with evidence.

Conclusion

Relevant and sustained evidence-informed practice requires a merging of research evidence, practice knowledge, and patients' perspectives (Sackett et al., 1996). This naturally extends to CHWs and their practice in which they should be able to both access and integrate evidence as well as to feedback their own experience and insights into the evidence base. In this framing, evidence-informed practice becomes yet another way in which workplace-based learning and development can take place. While currently systems and tools for EIDM, such as evidence maps, are not equipped to embed a learning and mentoring element into them, this seems to hold large future potential for CHWs. And, from an ethical perspective, there is a strong moral imperative for EIDM to become a less technical and more inclusive practice—which can then combine the more effective and equitable provision of healthcare practices by CHWs with the empowerment of CHWs as healthcare professionals.

Acknowledgements

The work presented in this chapter has been co-developed and supported by colleagues at the Africa Centre for Evidence, University of Johannesburg led by Prof. Ruth Stewart and by colleagues in the research unit of South Africa's National Department of Planning Monitoring and Evaluation led by Harsha Dayal.

References

Adichie, C. (2016). *The Danger of a Single Story*. Available from: https://www.ethos3.com/2016/04/3-lessons-from-chimamanda-ngozi-adichies-the-danger-of-a-single-story/

Chalmers, I. (2005). If evidence-informed policy works in practice, does it matter if it doesn't work in theory? *Evidence & Policy: A Journal of Research, Debate and Practice*, 1(2), 227–242.

Chalmers, I. & Glasziou, P. (2009). Avoidable waste in the production and reporting of research evidence. *Lancet*, 374(9683), 86–89.

Cochrane (2020). *Our Logo Tells a Story*. Available from: https://www.cochrane.org/about-us/difference-we-make.

Dayal, D. (2019). *Responding to Demand Side Evidence Needs and Ensuring Relevance. A Collaborative Model from South Africa*. Keynote presentation at the Qualitative Evidence Synthesis Symposium, Brazil, 9–11 October.

Dayal, D. & Langer, L. (2016). *Policy-relevant Evidence Maps: A Departmental Guidance Note*. Pretoria, DPME.

Department of Planning, Monitoring and Evaluation (DPME) (2016). *Socio-Economic Impact Assessment System (SEIAS). Final Impact Assessment Template (Phase 2) On Competition Amendment Bill*. Pretoria, DPME.

Department of Planning, Monitoring and Evaluation (DPME) (2020). *An Evidence Map on the National Health Insurance Bill*. DPME: Pretoria, South Africa.

Dixon-Woods, M., Agarwal, S., Jones, D., Young, B., & Sutton, A. (2005). Synthesising qualitative and quantitative evidence: A review of possible methods. *Journal of Health Services Research & Policy*, 10(1), 45–53.

Gilmore, B. & McAuliffe, E. (2013). Effectiveness of community health workers delivering preventive interventions for maternal and child health in low- and middle-income countries: A systematic review. *BMC Public Health*, 13(1), 847.

Glenton, C., Colvin, C.J., Carlsen, B., Swartz, A., Lewin, S., Noyes, J., & Rashidian, A. (2013). Barriers and facilitators to the implementation of lay health worker programmes to improve access to maternal and child health: A qualitative evidence synthesis. *Cochrane Database of Systematic Reviews*, (10), CD010414.

Gough, D., Oliver, S., & Thomas, J. (Eds) (2017). *An introduction to systematic reviews*. London, Sage.

Gough, D. & White, H. (2018). *Evidence standards and evidence claims in web based research portals*. London: Centre for Homelessness Impact. Accessed: https://eppi.ioe.ac.uk/cms/Default.aspx?tabid=3743

Greenhalgh, T. & Peacock, R. (2005). Effectiveness and efficiency of search methods in systematic reviews of complex evidence: Audit of primary sources. *British Medical Journal*, 331(7524), 1064–1065.

Haddaway, N.R. & Crowe, S. (2017). *Stakeholder Engagement in Environmental Evidence Synthesis*. Stockholm, Mistra EviEM.

Higgins, J.P. & Green, S. (Eds) (2011). *Cochrane Handbook for Systematic Reviews of Interventions* (Vol. 4). New York, John Wiley & Sons.

Kraemer-Mbula, E. & Nduku, P. (2019). *An Evidence Map of Innovation and Inclusive Industrialisation*. Johannesburg, University of Johannesburg.

Langer, L. & Stewart, R. (2014.) What have we learned from the application of systematic review methodology in international development?—a thematic overview. *Journal of Development Effectiveness*, 6(3), 236–248.

Langer, L. (2019). *Prioritising Demand Side Evidence Needs and Ensuring Relevance. A Collaborative Model from South Africa*. Keynote presentation at the Qualitative Evidence Synthesis Symposium. Brazil, 9–11 October.

Langer, L., Tripney, J., & Gough, D.A. (2016). *The Science of Using Science: Researching the Use of Research Evidence in Decision-making*. London, UCL Institute of Education, EPPI-Centre.

Lewin, S., Munabi-Babigumira, S., Glenton, C., Daniels, K., Bosch-Capblanch, X., Van Wyk, B.E., Odgaard-Jensen, J., Johansen, M., Aja, G.N., Zwarenstein, M., & Scheel, I.B. (2010). Lay health workers in primary and community health care for maternal and child health and the management of infectious diseases. *Cochrane Database of Systematic Reviews*, (3).

Miake-Lye, I.M., Hempel, S., Shanman, R., & Shekelle, P.G. (2016). What is an evidence map? A systematic review of published evidence maps and their definitions, methods, and products. *Systematic Reviews*, 5(1), 28.

Mijumbi-Deve, R. & Sewankambo, N.K. (2018). A process evaluation to assess contextual factors associated with the uptake of a rapid response service to support health systems' decision-making in Uganda. *International Journal of Health Policy and Management*, 6(10), 561.

Mijumbi-Deve, R., Rosenbaum, S.E., Oxman, A.D., Lavis, J.N., & Sewankambo, N.K. (2017). Policymaker experiences with rapid response briefs to address health-system and technology questions in Uganda. *Health Research Policy and Systems*, 15(1), 3.

Mwai, G.W., Mburu, G., Torpey, K., Frost, P., Ford, N., & Seeley, J. (2013). Role and outcomes of community health workers in HIV care in sub-Saharan Africa: A systematic review. *Journal of the International AIDS Society*, 16(1), 18586.

Nutley, S.M., Walter, I., & Davies, H.T. (2007). *Using Evidence: How Research Can Inform Public Services*. Bristol, Policy Press.

Nyqvist, M., Guariso, A., Svensson, J., & Yanagizawa-Drott, D. (2019). Reducing child mortality in the last mile: Experimental evidence on community health promoters in Uganda. *American Economic Journal: Applied Economics*, 11(3), 155–192.

Oakley, A. (2000). *Experiments in Knowing*. Cambridge, Polity Press.

O'Donovan, J., O'Donovan, C., Kuhn, I., Sachs, S.E., & Winters, N. (2018). Ongoing training of community health workers in low-income and middle-income countries: A systematic scoping review of the literature. *BMJ Open*, 8(4), e021467.

Oliver, S. (2014). Advantages of concurrent preparation and reporting of systematic reviews of quantitative and qualitative evidence. *Journal of the Royal Society of Medicine*, 108(3), 108–111.

Parkhurst, J. (2017). *The Politics of Evidence: From Evidence-based Policy to the Good Governance of Evidence*. Abingdon, Routledge.

Pawson, R. (2006). *Evidence-Based Policy: A Realist Perspective*. London, Sage.

Petticrew, M. & Roberts, H. (2006). *Systematic Reviews in the Social Sciences: A Practical Guide*. New York, John Wiley & Sons.

Sackett, D.L., Rosenberg, W.M., Gray, J.M., Haynes, R.B., & Richardson, W.S. (1996). Evidence-based medicine: What it is and what it isn't. *British Medical Journal*, 313(7050), 169–171.

Snilstveit, B., Vojtkova, M., Bhavsar, A., & Gaarder, M. (2013). *Evidence Gap Maps—a Tool for Promoting Evidence-Informed Policy and Prioritizing Future Research*. Washington DC, World Bank.

Snilstveit, B., Vojtkova, M., Bhavsar, A., Stevenson, J., & Gaarder, M. (2016). Evidence & gap maps: A tool for promoting evidence informed policy and strategic research agendas. *Journal of Clinical Epidemiology*, 79, 120–129.

Stewart, R. (2014). Changing the world one systematic review at a time: A new development methodology for making a difference. *Development Southern Africa*, 31(4), 581–590.

Stewart, R., Dayal, H., & Langer, L. (2017). Terminology and tensions within evidence-informed decision-making in South Africa over a 15-year period. *Research for All*, 1(2), 252–264.

Stewart, R., Langer, L., & Erasmus, Y. (2018). An integrated model for increasing the use of evidence by decision-makers for improved development. *Development Southern Africa*, 36(5), 1–16.

Stewart, R., Dayal, H., Langer, L., & Van Rooyen, C. (2019). The evidence ecosystem in South Africa: Growing resilience and institutionalisation of evidence use. *Palgrave Communications*, 5(1), 1–12.

Suthar, A.B. & Bärnighausen, T. (2017). Antiretroviral therapy and population mortality: Leveraging routine national data to advance policy. *PLoS Medicine*, 14(12), e1002469.

Tricco, A.C., Langlois, E.V., & Straus, S.E. (Eds) (2017). *Rapid Reviews to Strengthen Health Policy and Systems: A Practical Guide*. Geneva, World Health Organization.

Van Ginneken, N., Tharyan, P., Lewin, S., Rao, G.N., Meera, S.M., Pian, J., et al. (2013). Non-specialist health worker interventions for the care of mental, neurological and substance-abuse disorders in low-and middle-income countries. *Cochrane Database of Systematic Reviews*, 19(11), CD009149.

Van Rooyen, C., Chen, S., Ncube, L., Huang, K., Tannous, N., & Langer, L. (2021). A scoping review of rapid synthesis services to support evidence-informed decision-making. *Evidence & Policy*. Forthcoming.

Vouking, M.Z., Takougang, I., Mbam, L.M., Mbuagbaw, L., Tadenfok, C.N., & Tamo, C.V. (2013). The contribution of community health workers to the control of Buruli ulcer in the Ngoantet area, Cameroon. *Pan African Medical Journal*, 16(1).

Weyrauch, V. (2016). *Knowledge into Policy: Going Beyond Context Matters*. Available from: http://www.politicsandideas.org/wp-content/uploads/2016/07/Going-beyond-context-matters-Framework_PI.compressed.pdf

Winters, N., Langer, L., Nduku, P., Robson, J., O'Donovan, J., Maulik, P., et al. (2019). Using mobile technologies to support the training of community health workers in low-income and middle-income countries: Mapping the evidence. *BMJ Global Health*, 4(4), e001421.

World Health Organization (2018). *WHO Guideline on Health Policy and System Support to Optimize Community Health Worker Programmes*. Geneva, World Health Organization.

10

Methods of Evaluation of Community Health Worker Training

Theory and Practice

Celia Brown

Introduction: Why Do We Need to Evaluate CHW Training?

'Every element of the [training] programme design has an impact on the outcome and effectiveness of the training'

Reproduced with permission from Saravanan, S., Turrell, G., Johnson, H. et al, Re-examining authoritative knowledge in the design and content of a TBA training in India. *Midwifery*, **28(1): 120–130. Copyright © 2011 Elsevier Ltd. All rights reserved.**

A 2014 review of over one hundred documents related to the training of CHWs in sub-Saharan Africa and South Asia concluded that: 'The literature points to a need for mandatory, consistent evaluation of training programs' (Redick & Dini, 2014, p. v). Why is such evaluation important? The 'big picture' answer to this question is that without effective training, CHWs will not be able to maximize their potential as health workers, and may even be unsafe (Taylor et al., 2018). CHW programme providers therefore need to be able to provide evidence that their training is effective in preparing CHWs for their roles (or in maintaining or enhancing their knowledge and skills over time). This is particularly important given that many CHWs have limited initial training periods—two to three weeks is not uncommon (Olaniran, et al., 2017). Underpinning this big picture answer is the awareness that training eats into the CHW programme budget, so any training provided needs to make the best use of the scarce resources available. There are many modifiable components of CHW training which have an impact on both cost and effectiveness (e.g. length, class size, and pedagogy): understanding these impacts to enable the cost-effective use of the scarce resources requires that the training is evaluated.

Before we begin, it is important to define what we mean by 'evaluation' and how it differs from 'monitoring'. The latter is the process of determining whether the training took place as intended: did everyone (trainers and trainees) show up? Was the planned

Celia Brown, *Methods of Evaluation of Community Health Worker Training* In: *Training for Community Health.* Edited by: Anne Geniets, James O'Donovan, Laura Hakimi, and Niall Winters, Oxford University Press. © Oxford University Press 2021. DOI: 10.1093/oso/9780198866244.003.0010

content delivered using the planned methods? Was the quality of the training satisfactory? Were trainees satisfied with the training? The former, meanwhile, is the process of determining whether the intended outcomes of the training were met (and also, perhaps, why or why not): generally this is the extent to which knowledge and/or skills improved. These two concepts of monitoring and evaluation are clearly related—if the training did not take place as intended, it is unlikely to be effective.

Developing a Logic Model

A logic model is a step-by-step description of an intervention. It is 'logical' in the sense that the steps are in temporal order: the model shows what needs to happen, and in what order, for an intervention to be effective. Logic models (or an equivalent) should be developed by those designing interventions but are mentioned here because they are also helpful in the design of evaluations of interventions. It may seem unnecessary to formally develop a logic model by thinking through the process—or causal chain—by which the provision of training to CHWs will improve their knowledge and/or skills and have the intended positive impact on patient care and health outcomes. But not all training is sufficiently effective. For example, in one study CHWs across four countries were trained in the assessment of cardiovascular risk (Gaziano et al., 2015). CHWs' competence was assessed using written and skills tests as well as by observations during supervised practice. Of the 68 CHWs trained, only 42 (62%) were deemed sufficiently competent to perform cardiovascular assessments in the field. If there are no, or insufficient, discernible effects of the training on outcomes, then it is important to ask why this was the case so that appropriate changes can be made. (An alternative explanation could be that the CHWs were poorly selected for their role; so it may also be important to examine selection criteria and processes. Thus, including any 'prerequisites' to training in the logic model is recommended.)

A logic model gives us the basis for identifying *barriers and facilitators* to effectiveness, which will help us explain why the training was or was not effective. Others have highlighted the importance of thinking in this way; for example Saravanan et al. note that while previous training of traditional birth attendants (TBAs) in India was not effective, there was no understanding as to why this was the case, such that it was not possible to determine how the training should be improved (Saravanan et al., 2012). The development of a logic model may also be an intervention in itself, for it helps those designing training identify what needs to happen for the training to be effective and brings these issues to the forefront of their minds during the design phase.

There is existing guidance on the development of logic models (Kneale et al., 2015); an example of applying a modified form of this approach for interventions to reduce the rate of diagnostic errors is presented by Kletter et al. (Kletter et al., 2018). For the logic models developed by Kletter and colleagues for interventions using education and feedback, the underlying theory for many of the steps included was based on the Kirkpatrick hierarchy of outcomes of educational interventions (Kirkpatrick, 1967).

This hierarchy shows how the provision of training can result in measurable outcomes at up to five ascending levels: participation, positive trainee reactions, learning by trainees, changes in the behaviour of trainees (the application of learning), and finally the desired results (in this case improved health). We now apply this approach to develop an illustrative logic model for a CHW training course on using rapid diagnostic tests (RDT) for malaria, a task undertaken by many CHWs. The provision of training for this task is particularly important due to safety concerns with the use of taking blood samples and the appropriate use of artemisinin combination therapy; but such training can be effective, and superior to the use of printed instructions and job aids alone (Harvey et al., 2008; Counihan et al., 2012). The ultimate outcomes of the training—for the CHW and their programme—would be that a CHW is able to administer an RDT correctly, interpret the results, refer patients for treatment if necessary, and, if appropriate, assist patients to attend for treatment and encourage them to complete their course of treatment. But what steps are necessary between the decision to provide training and achieving these outcomes? A potential logic model is shown in Figure 10.1. Each stage in the logic model is a potential point at which training could fail to achieve its intended outcomes. An end point at each stage could therefore be measured as part of the evaluation; commonly used end points are shown in bold in Figure 10.1 (see section End Points/Outcomes and Measurements in this chapter for further details). By thinking through the model—a process known as pre-implementation evaluation (Brown et al., 2008a)—possible ways, or mechanisms, in which effectiveness could 'flow out' of the model can be identified and several example flows have been added to Figure 10.1. These include a poor match of the level of the training with CHWs' existing literacy and skills, a failure to support attendance by not paying travel costs or a *per diem* to compensate for lost earnings (particularly for volunteer CHWs), an uninteresting format causing CHWs to become disengaged, and not ensuring an adequate supply chain of essential equipment such as RDTs and gloves. Exploring these mechanisms in an evaluation may require qualitative approaches in a mixed methods design; and as we will see in section Mixed Methods Evaluations, these should be planned in advance of implementation wherever possible.

Choosing a Study Design

The guiding principle for choosing a study design is to use the design that would provide the strongest evidence of causality for the research question being addressed, providing it is ethical and practical to do so. Our overarching research question would be: 'Is the CHW training provided effective?' To answer this question we not only need to measure the chosen end -point(s)/outcome(s) after the provision of training (see section End Points/Outcomes and Measurements in this chapter), but we also need to know (or be able to estimate) what those measurements would have been in the absence of the provision of training; in other words, what the *counterfactual* would have

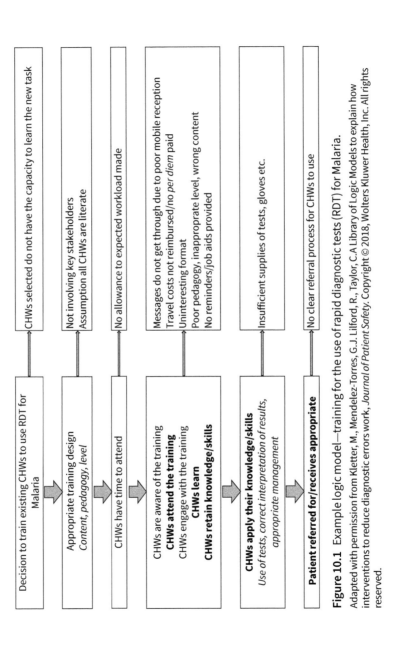

Figure 10.1 Example logic model—training for the use of rapid diagnostic tests (RDT) for Malaria.

Adapted with permission from Kletter, M., Mendelez-Torres, G.J. Lilford, R., Taylor, C.A Library of Logic Models to explain how interventions to reduce diagnostic errors work, *Journal of Patient Safety*. Copyright © 2018, Wolters Kluwer Health, Inc. All rights reserved.

Box 10.1 Differences in differences

	Control group	Intervention group
Before training	A	B
After training	C	D
Differences in differences:	(D – B) – (C – A)	

The difference between the change in outcomes in the intervention group and the change in outcomes in the control group.

been. There are two ways of obtaining information about the counterfactual to CHW training: using measurements taken before the training and/or using measurements taken from a comparable control group of CHWs who did not receive the training (or, if we wished to compare two forms of training, from CHWs who received a different form of training). Studies in epistemology would tell us that the strongest study design would be to randomly allocate CHWs to the intervention and control groups (a randomized controlled trial, or RCT) *and* to take before-and-after measurements (Brown et al., 2008b). This would enable calculation of *effect sizes*[1] as 'differences in differences' (Box 10.1); an approach which usually minimizes bias (Brown et al., 2008b). Using before-and-after measurements alone, without a control group, is a relatively weak study design, as it is difficult to attribute causality to the intervention when other influences on outcomes—such as the implementation of a new national policy or even a change in the weather—could be occurring simultaneously, and when *regression to the mean*[2] could be a problem. Selection bias, when the CHWs most likely to benefit from the training are selected to participate in the evaluation, is also a possibility.

However, the use of before-training measurements of knowledge and/or skill may result in bias due to 'question behaviour effects', because the assessment of knowledge/skill itself acts as an intervention (McCambridge, 2015). Those who have taken the initial assessment but not received the training may become more 'test-wise'. The same may occur for those who have received the intervention, but these individuals may also

---

[1] An *effect size* is a quantitative assessment of the extent of the change in outcomes occurring as a result of training. Effect sizes are standardized to enable comparisons between different interventions to be made. For example, for a simple post-training comparison of intervention and control groups, the absolute difference in outcomes (assuming a continuous, normally distributed outcome) is denominated on the pooled standard deviation (i.e. (mean score intervention – mean score control)/pooled standard deviation).

[2] *Regression to the mean* is best described with an example. Patients with a high blood pressure reading are recruited into a study to evaluate the effectiveness of a lifestyle intervention on reducing blood pressure. On a follow-up reading, the mean blood pressure in the intervention group has fallen considerably, so it appears the intervention has been effective. However, blood pressure readings are known to fluctuate, so it is likely that those selected into the study with a high baseline measurement would have had a lower measurement at follow-up in the absence of an intervention: their blood pressure would have regressed to the mean.

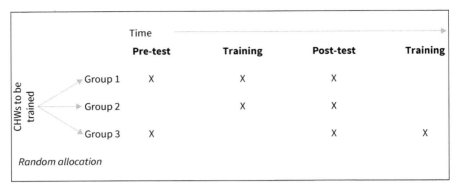

Figure 10.2 Suggested modified Solomon design for evaluation of CHW training.

be 'cued' by the content of the original assessment and focus on these curriculum areas during the training in order to improve their performance. As a result, the effect size for the training is likely to be biased. A Modified Solomon study design combines the tenets of randomization with partial before-and-after measurements to provide a solution to this problem (Solomon, 1949), providing that it is possible to delay providing training to one third of the CHWs and ethical to make before-training measurements. CHWs are randomized into three groups, as shown in Figure 10.2[3]. We used a different modification to the Solomon design in a formative evaluation of a CHW training course in KwaZulu Natal in South Africa (Plowright et al., 2018). For one of the two cohorts we found a significant improvement in written test scores for the group that had not received the intervention, which even seemed too great an improvement to attribute to participants gaining 'test-wiseness' alone. Follow-up qualitative work enabled us to understand this effect: the CHWs in the 'delayed training' group were not confident that they would receive the training as promised (and as was delivered) because they had been let down in the past. They therefore sought out other means of learning the material covered in the initial assessment, for example by asking their supervisors.

There are also some circumstances in which the use of an RCT (Modified Solomon) with before-and-after measurements is not ethical or practical, and where an alternative study design is required. These circumstances are as follows:

- When there is a lack of *equipoise*. This is a key ethical requirement for conducting an RCT (Lilford & Jackson, 1995). Equipoise exists when there is

---

[3] We have assumed that it is necessary to train all CHWs (in one way or another) and therefore we have not included the fourth group from the original Solomon Design, which did not receive training. In an ideal world, the training would not be given (in its current form) to those in Modified Solomon Group 3 unless it was shown to be effective, but this may also be logistically difficult or create issues in relation to perceived fairness, particularly if longer-term outcomes are being measured (see section End Points/Outcomes and Measurements in this chapter). This Modified Solomon Design is therefore similar to a delayed implementation RCT but the baseline (pre-test) is not administered to those in one group.

genuine uncertainty about which course of action should be taken: for example if a new drug is more effective than the current treatment. If society 'knows' that one treatment is superior to another, then research to compare the two is unethical because the research would put participants at unnecessary risk of harm. A CHW programme team in this situation should reconsider what they are trying to evaluate and why.

- When the end points to be measured include outcomes such as quality of care and CHWs have not previously been trained in the content area. Before training measurements and after training measurements for a no training control group (Modified Solomon Group 3) would not be ethical because it could be dangerous to allow untrained CHWs to be deployed to work with patients. An RCT with measurements after training only would be appropriate in this situation if the comparator is a different approach to training rather than no training; otherwise it would only be possible to use surrogate outcomes such as a written test (see section End Points/Outcomes and Measurements' in this chapter).

- When it would be impractical or too expensive to delay training for any CHWs and there is no opportunity to compare two approaches to training: an uncontrolled before-and-after study may be the only possible study design in this situation, and it may only be possible to measure surrogate outcomes.

Clearly, choosing the strongest study design that is feasible and ethical requires careful consideration by an evaluation team. Box 10.2 gives two examples of existing evaluations of CHW training using different study designs.

We have yet to consider the *unit* of allocation in evaluations of CHW training that include a control group (Modified Solomon Group 3). It may be possible to allocate individual CHWs to either the intervention or control group, particularly if CHWs tend to work alone in their own villages. However, if CHWs are attached to health centres, for example, it may be necessary to allocate all CHWs attached to one health centre to the same study group (intervention or control). This is for two reasons. The first is the practicality of having to run two separate trainings at a single health centre. The second is the epistemological problem of contamination. The CHWs who work together are likely to talk amongst themselves; word of the training being received by some may spread to those allocated to the control group, who may seek out their own learning and/or attend the training as if they were in the intervention group. CHW programme providers may also find it challenging to justify why only some CHWs are being trained (even if the disparity is only temporary). When CHWs are allocated in groups (e.g. by health centre) rather than as individuals, then this is known as a *cluster* design, with each group forming one cluster. Considerable care is required when undertaking—and particularly when analysing the data from—cluster studies, because of the existence of *intra-cluster correlations*: individual CHWs within each cluster are likely to be more similar to CHWs from their own cluster than to CHWs from other clusters. Donner and Klar provide an excellent introduction to cluster studies in their book (Donner & Klar, 2000).

Box 10.2 Examples of evaluations of CHW training using different study designs

Before-and-after study design (Msisuka et al., 2011)

Twenty-five lay HIV counsellors in Zambia were given two days of refresher training. Written and skills tests (comprising 25 true/false questions and testing 10 blood samples respectively) were completed by the CHWs before and after the training in order to evaluate the effectiveness of the training. While mean scores on the written test increased from 79% to 95%, there was no change in the skills assessment results, because performance before the training was almost perfect (there was no 'headroom' for improvement). Question behaviour effects, in terms of participants being 'cued' to the content of the written test during the training, were a distinct possibility and may have biased the after-training scores upwards. In addition, the participants were selected as those 'most active' from each health facility, and such selection bias means the results may not be generalizable to the population of lay counsellors (a problem acknowledged by the authors).

Non-randomized study design with after-training measurements (Harvey et al., 2008)

Seventy-nine CHWs were allocated to one of three groups given different levels of training in how to use RDT for malaria: access to the manufacturer's instructions only, a job aid, and a three-hour training session plus the job aid. The method used to allocate CHWs to the three groups was not fully described, so allocation bias could affect the results. CHWs were assessed after the provision of these materials on their ability to conduct RDT safely and to interpret the results of such tests correctly. Because using RDT was a new procedure for CHWs, assessments were only undertaken following the training; this also had the advantage of mitigating bias due to question behaviour effects. CHWs who received the training and had access to the job aid performed better than CHWs in the other two groups, suggesting that the training was effective.

One further potential study design that may be appropriate if training is to be rolled-out across groups/clusters of CHWs over time is the cluster randomized stepped wedge design (Brown & Lilford, 2006; Taljaard et al., 2015). It is not always possible to train all CHWs within a programme at once, particularly if CHWs are located across a wide geographical area or if there are limitations on class size. In a cluster stepped wedge design, the order in which each group (or cluster) of CHWs receives the training is determined at random, but, by the end of the roll-out period, all CHWs will have received the training, so there are no ethical issues with regards to withholding training from some CHWs. However, this approach does mean that there should be sufficient a priori evidence that the training is effective. Determining the order of roll-out at random is also a fair so-lution when it must be staggered. The stepped wedge design is most feasible when the end points to be measured use routinely-collected data, so that such data can be collected at every time period (i.e. when each new cluster receives training) without considerable additional expense. As such data are likely to include CHW activity data, this design may only be ethical for refresher training rather than ini-tial training. The Partners in Health CHW programme team in Neno, Malawi, are using a cluster randomized stepped wedge design to evaluate a new approach to CHW programme delivery across the entire district, which involves re-training all existing and some newly-recruited CHWs in the new *household model* of care (Dunbar et al., 2018).

As we have seen, the choice of study design turns, in part, on what outcomes, or end points are to be measured in the evaluation, and it is to this issue that we now turn.

End Points/Outcomes and Measurement

What do we expect to change as a result of the provision of training to CHWs? Ideally, we would want to see that the health of CHWs' patients had improved. However, patients' health may not be the most appropriate end point, or outcome measure in an evaluation of CHW training. In the section Developing a Logic Model above, we used the Kirkpatrick hierarchy of outcomes (Kirkpatrick, 1967) to help us de-velop a logic model describing how training could have an impact on the desired patient-level outcomes. The different steps in a logic model each present an oppor-tunity for measuring the effectiveness of training. The outcomes above (occurring before) patient-level health outcomes in the logic model are collectively known as surrogate outcomes (Brown et al., 2008c). In this section, we consider five poten-tial outcomes to help those planning an evaluation decide which one(s) to measure. When making this decision, it is useful to bear in mind the key intended objective of the training (which is likely to be one of the steps in the logic model) and to focus efforts on measuring the outcome closest to this step (e.g. the relevant outcome in bold in Figure 10.1). Where possible, the measurement of multiple outcomes is re-commended, but trade-offs between optimal evaluation design, cost and feasibility often have to be made.

Tests of CHWs' Knowledge

The majority of existing evaluations of CHW training include a written post-training assessment of CHWs' knowledge of the content area of the training; oral tests may also be used, perhaps where CHW literacy levels are low (e.g. Agrawal et al., 2011). The questions used in these tests can take a number of forms: true/false, multiple choice, fill-in-the-blank, or a mixture of these (and others); (see e.g. Msisuka et al., 2011; O'Donovan et al., 2018; Plowright et al., 2018; Taylor et al., 2018). Such tests can be administered fairly easily and at low cost. However, knowledge tests have two key weaknesses. The first is that the results of an evaluation based on test scores rely on the quality of the test, particularly in terms of its immediate validity and reliability (Box 10.3). The second is that—as a surrogate outcome—tests of knowledge are only useful if they also have *predictive validity*. Scores on the test need to be a good proxy for CHWs' on-the-job performance and ultimately, health outcomes. One study undertaken with Anganwadi workers in India does suggest a strong positive relationship between CHWs' knowledge regarding antenatal care and the antenatal home visit coverage and effectiveness achieved (Agrawal et al., 2011). However such a positive relationship should not always be assumed to exist.

Box 10.3 Assessing the assessment

The *validity* of a test is the extent to which it measures what it is intended to measure, at an appropriate level. The content of a test should be representative of the entire training curriculum (which itself should be developed based on an analysis of what CHWs need to know, and be able to do). The test also needs to be set at an appropriate level for the CHWs who will be taking it. It is all too easy to set a test where what is being assessed is literacy, rather than job-related knowledge. Key threats to validity include only including questions on content areas that are easy to assess, not reviewing the draft test against the curriculum, and using easy-to-mark test formats that encourage guessing and are not representative of real life. True/false and multiple choice questions both fall into this category. Drawing from a study of assessment in medical education, 'patients do not walk into the clinic saying "I have one of these five diagnoses. Which do you think is most likely?"' (Surry et al., 2017).

The *reliability* of a test is the extent to which it produces consistent results both within itself and over time (Wass et al., 2001). If different questions from the 'pool' of all potential questions that could have been included been asked, would CHWs obtain a similar score? If CHWs sat the same test the next day (without learning anything from taking the first test), would they obtain a similar score? If the answer to either question is no, then the test may not be sufficiently reliable. A key threat to reliability is the length of the test: the more questions that are included, the greater the content that can be assessed and thus the less likely it is that the test only includes questions that an individual CHW does or does not know the answer to. We've probably all come out of exams celebrating that only what we had revised had come up, or moaning because what we had revised had not come up at all. Had those exams been longer, the proportion of the content that we had revised would be about the same as the proportion of that content in the exam.

In Vitro Tests of CHW Skills

It is often possible to set up post-training skills tests for CHWs, in which CHWs complete the tasks required of them as a CHW but in a simulated setting, so there is no risk of patient harm. Examples include taking anthropometric measurements (Gaziano et al., 2015), interpreting RDT test results (Harvey et al., 2008), and using video-based scenarios to assess children for pneumonia (O'Donovan et al., 2018). Such tests are more akin to 'real life' than knowledge tests, so are likely to have higher predictive validity, although it is still essential to consider the validity and reliability of such skills tests.

In Vivo Assessment of CHW On-The-Job Performance

Assessing the on-the-job performance of CHWs is potentially the optimal outcome measure for evaluating training, as it provides good validity and can be measured with much better precision than patient health outcomes (see below). As such, on-the-job performance has been used in various studies evaluating CHW training (e.g. Uzochukwu et al., 2008; Lopes et al., 2014). However, as noted in the section Choosing a Study Design in this chapter, it would not be ethical to use in vivo assessments on a new content area before training is provided. Perhaps the 'gold standard' approach to determining the quality of care provided by a CHW is direct observation followed by independent re-examination by a clinician (Cardemil et al., 2012), but this is particularly resource intensive. Concurrent direct observation by a trained observer only is a common approach, but again is resource intensive. Hawthorne effects may occur when direct observation is used, with CHWs trying to ensure they provide optimal care because they are being observed. One solution is to discard the first set of observations, because participants in most studies tend to 'forget' they are being observed over time. A final consideration is the number of cases/patients that should be included: in the study Uzochukwu et al., consultations with less than two sick children per health worker were observed (Uzochukwu et al., 2008), and this is unlikely to be sufficient to enable reliable measurements of health worker performance to be made.

Routine CHW Activity Data

An easily accessible outcome measure is the routine data collected as part of implementation of the CHW programme itself. Mobile platforms such as Medic enable the timely collection of data about household visits and care provided, for example, at no cost to the evaluation team. However, routine data may not be 'fit for purpose' for evaluating CHW training—for example, they may consider the *amount* of activity undertaken, but not the *quality* of such activity, or whether the learning from the training is being applied. Nevertheless, it is always worth reviewing what routine data are available, because they could form part of a suite of outcome measures which together can tell a powerful story about the effectiveness of CHW training. For example, knowing that CHWs are undertaking RDTs for malaria having been trained to do so for the first time shows at least that the training is being put into practice.

Patient-Level Health Outcomes

The final possible outcome considered in this section is patient health. In some cases, it may be possible to collect data on mortality, potentially using routine data. Health-related quality of life could be measured using general scales such as the EQ-5D (see: https://euroqol.org/), or, if the training is for a specific health/disease area, by using a disease-specific scale. However, not all scales have been validated for all populations, so careful consideration of which one(s) to use is required. The collection of health outcome data may present logistical challenges: ideally collection would be undertaken by an independent data collector who is blinded to the CHW's training status, which would require additional household visits. Distal outcomes such as mortality and health-related quality of life can be affected by many things and the proportionate influence of CHW training is likely to be very small. As explained below, it would be necessary to obtain data from a very large sample of the population, adding to feasibility constraints.

When to Measure Outcomes in Relation to the Training

The most common time to measure outcomes is immediately following the provision of training. This reduces the likelihood of other influences, such as subsequent CHW supervisions, biasing the results, but what has been learned during a training course may not be retained for long enough to have a lasting effect on patient health. Therefore repeated measurements of outcomes are encouraged where it is feasible to do so. While some studies looking at longer-term retention of knowledge have shown good retention over 12 (Counihan et al., 2012) and 18 months (Gobezayehu et al., 2014), others highlight the need for regular refresher training in order to maintain initial gains (Shrivastava & Shrivastava, 2012).

Sample Size, Precision, and Sampling

There are two components to the question of sample size: (1) how many CHWs to include in a research or evaluation study and (2) how many assessment items (e.g. test questions or patient observations) to include. It may seem that more of both is better: holding all else constant, the *precision* of any statistical estimate of effectiveness will increase with the sample size and we have already seen how the reliability of an assessment tool is positively influenced by sample size. But evaluation is not cost free and if the training turns out to be ineffective then patient health could be jeopardized. In a clinical trial of a new drug, it is important to strike the right balance between trial cost, getting a precise estimate of effectiveness, and minimizing the number of participants who could be harmed. The same principles apply to evaluations of CHW training. A further consideration is the size of the effect that is being sought: to what extent should the training improve outcomes? The larger the size of the effect being sought, the smaller the sample size can be (in terms of achieving statistical precision), because the likelihood of a large effect occurring by chance alone is much lower than that of a small effect. Arguably we would expect training to have a relatively large effect on knowledge test scores, but relatively smaller effects as the outcome measure(s) become more distal from the training: patient health outcomes can be affected by a vast number of factors, of which CHW training is only one.

In a two-group comparison with a normally distributed outcome such as knowledge test or quality of care scores, we have seen that the size of the difference in scores between the groups can be shown using the *effect size*. Cohen suggested that a small effect size would be around 0.2 standard deviations, a medium effect size 0.5, and a large effect size 0.8 (Cohen, 1988). To have 80% statistical power to detect an effect size of 0.2 at the standard critical p-value of 0.05 in a two-group comparison would require a total of 788 CHWs. For a large effect size (0.8), this would fall to 52 CHWs. While statistical sample size calculations should be used to guide theoretical sample size decisions, other factors, such as any anticipated attrition and the *educational significance* of the effect size, also need to be considered. In a formative evaluation of CHW training in South Africa, Plowright and colleagues found post-test scores had an overall mean of around 36/56 (64%) and a standard deviation of 6 marks (Plowright et al., 2018). A small effect size of 0.2 standard deviations would be a difference in mean scores of 1.2 marks (2 percentage points) and a large effect size of 0.8 standard deviations 4.8 marks (9 percentage points). Whether training that only increases knowledge test scores by 2 percentage points would be value for money is a key question here.

If a sample of CHWs (and, potentially, of CHWs' patients) are to be recruited for the evaluation, a related question is *how* the CHWs should be selected. Of course, all participants need to consent to being included in the evaluation, but care is needed to avoid selection bias, where the CHWs and/or patients included are systematically different to those who are not. Selection bias may rise if selection is based on literacy, proximity to a health centre, or length of service, for example. Random selection from the pool of CHWs and their patients should be used wherever possible.

Mixed Methods Evaluations

In previous sections we focused on study designs and outcomes/end points for quantitative research methods; yet in the first section of this chapter we noted the importance of a mixed methods design to enable evaluators to consider *why* a training intervention had the level of effectiveness found in the quantitative analysis. We therefore fill in the gap in this section. The potential flows out of the logic model give an indication as to what issues could be important to include in qualitative data collection. It is also important to explore *facilitators* to effectiveness as well as *barriers*; particularly if the training is to be repeated locally and also to share such findings with other CHW programme providers. Complementary qualitative approaches to data collection include interviews and/or focus groups with training providers, CHW participants and CHWs' patients. Such methods should be planned concurrently with any quantitative data collection, with thought given to who to include and how to recruit participants, as well as what approach to data collection and analysis to use. For example, interviewers and focus group facilitators need to be skilled in eliciting unbiased information from participants, and interview schedules or guides may need to be piloted in advance of formal data collection. There may also be unanticipated issues that impact on effectiveness, so in some situations *post-hoc* qualitative work may be required; even if such work is not appropriate for publication, it may still shed light on issues worthy of further study. Creswell and Plano-Clark's introductory text (Creswell & Clark, 2017) provides a useful starting point for those wanting to use a mixed methods approach to gain a better understanding of training effectiveness than could be achieved with one method alone (which in this chapter we have assumed to be quantitative). It is also important to plan how the results will be integrated across different methods, with possible approaches including 'follow the thread' or the 'Pillar Integration Process' (O'Cathain et al., 2010; Johnson et al., 2017). Both of these approaches provide a systematic way of seeking explanations for quantitative findings in the qualitative data. A further approach to using mixed methods to enhance CHW training would be to conduct preliminary qualitative work to identify CHWs' learning needs and to use the results to help design the training itself (see Plowright et al., 2018, where the research team was fortunate enough to obtain funding for intervention development to enable the preliminary qualitative work to be undertaken).

Other Considerations in Designing Evaluations of CHW Training

There are a number of other important factors that need to be considered when designing evaluations of CHW training, which are summarized below.

- Should you include a measure of participation rates and/or questionnaire to gauge CHWs' reactions to (or satisfaction with) the training? We have not considered such outcome measures in any detail, as they are more akin to monitoring and cannot provide an estimate of training effectiveness. They could, however, help to explain a lack of effectiveness, for example if CHWs reported being unable to attend or understand the training, or being disengaged with the activities.

- Have you ascertained the feasibility of your intended outcome measures? Are they acceptable to CHWs (and, if appropriate, their patients)? Can they be completed in a timely manner without increasing CHWs' workloads? What training is required for those using them (e.g. observers)? A pilot of your outcome measures is likely to be very informative.

- Can, or should you, include an economic evaluation? Other studies—albeit undertaken in different countries at different times—have estimated the cost of providing refresher training or continuing development (as opposed to initial training before deployment) to CHWs in the range of US$ 48–128 per CHW per day (Chin-Quee et al., 2013; Gaziano et al., 2015; Plowright et al., 2018), so it may be useful to consider how the cost of your own training compares (and why), bearing in mind differences in local price levels at the time of training and the 'intensity' of the training. An economic evaluation may be particularly helpful if you are comparing two different approaches to training and you want to determine if the more expensive approach is likely to be value for money.

- Do you need to obtain permissions to undertake the evaluation? If you want to publish the results you will need ethical approval, at least in the country where the research is taking place and, if the research team is located in another country, in their country too. Some countries also have national research councils which oversee all research, so the study will need to be registered once ethical approval is obtained. A randomized trial should also be registered, for example on https:// clinicaltrials.gov/.

- Have you considered how the data collected during the evaluation will be stored and processed? Any data about, or collected from, research participants must be stored securely and in line with national and/or international regulations, such as the EU General Data Protection Regulation (GDPR); see https://eugdpr.org. uk/. This is particularly pertinent for any identifying personal or sensitive data, including contact details and demographics. Any process of data entry, for example manual entry of test scores to a computerized database is subject to data entry errors, so it is important to think about how the accuracy of data entry will be checked.

- Do you have the appropriate in-house statistical expertise to help you plan the evaluation and subsequently undertake the data analysis? If not, it is worth seeking advice as early as possible, because involving a statistician at an early stage can help to prevent difficulties later on. The same rule applies for expertise in qualitative data collection and analysis.

- How will you ensure the safety of researchers/evaluators? Many organizations have a lone-worker policy, but even in teams researchers could be at risk in remote settings. The safety of CHWs is also critical, but attendance at training should be covered in existing CHW programme policies.

- When is it most appropriate to undertake training and evaluation? Variations in climate may mean that disease prevalence and the ability to travel are not constant throughout the year. For example, if training and evaluation are undertaken during the rainy season, would the same level of effectiveness be found if they were repeated in the dry season?
- It is good practice to provide sufficient detail about the training intervention so that it could be replicated elsewhere. To date, this has not always been the case for CHW training (Saravanan et al., 2012), and this has made it challenging to spread good practice (and prevent repetition of preventable flaws in training programme design). The Template for Intervention Description and Replication (Hoffmann et al., 2014) is a good starting point for what to include in such a description. A good analogy for such a description is whether you could follow a recipe from a recipe book and produce the same result as in the picture in the book.
- Likewise, there are now checklists available for almost all evaluation study designs to help guide the reporting or writing-up process (see http://www.equator-network.org/). Most journals now require a completed checklist for the appropriate study design to be submitted with articles for potential publication (and it is worth working through this while planning an evaluation to ensure all requirements have been or can be met). The data collected during an evaluation should also be published whenever possible (after being completely anonymized). Data repositories such as https://www.mendeley.com/ provide a platform for such data preservation and publication.
- Finally, it is just as important to publish results from evaluations when the training has not been as effective as it is to publish results when the training was effective. Hiding away negative results is one form of publication bias and prevents others from learning from your experiences when things did not go completely according to plan.

Conclusions

Evaluating CHW training is clearly an important activity; planning an evaluation concurrently with the training itself is encouraged (and may actually help identify potential issues with the training as planned). There is no 'one size fits all' approach to evaluation (Brown et al., 2008a) and the appropriate approach will depend on the existing evidence regarding the training planned, the intended audience for the evaluation and the resources available for the evaluation. However any approach can, and should be, undertaken systematically, as advocated by Redick and Dini (2014). Scrimping on any aspect of an evaluation may be a false economy if the implication is a large group of CHWs who are sub-optimally trained, but if the training proposed already has a solid and generalizable evidence base, the evaluation is for internal purposes only and the knowledge/skills being taught are 'low risk' (i.e. there is little risk of patient harm), then a simple before-and-after study may suffice. However, any opportunity to use random selection or allocation should be taken when it is possible to do so (Leigh, 2018). Regardless of the approach to evaluation chosen, using published guides to describe the training and writing-up the evaluation will help to guide these activities and may help to prevent '*if only...*' moments once the opportunity to design the evaluation and/or collect data has been lost.

References

Agrawal, P.K., Agrawal, S., Ahmed, S., Darmstadt, G.L., Williams, E.K., Rosen, H.E., et al. (2011). Effect of knowledge of community health workers on essential newborn health care: A study from rural India. *Health Policy & Planning*, 27(2), 115–126.

Brown, C., Hofer, T., Johal, A., Thomson, R., Nicholl, J., Franklin, B., et al. (2008a). An epistemology of patient safety research: A framework for study design and interpretation. Part 4. One size does not fit all. *Quality & Safety in Health Care*, 17. doi:10.1136/qshc.2007.023663

Brown, C., Hofer, T., Johal, A., Thomson, R., Nicholl, J., Franklin, B., et al. (2008b). An epistemology of patient safety research: A framework for study design and interpretation. Part 2. Study design. *Quality and Safety in Health Care*, 17(3), 163–169.

Brown, C., Hofer, T., Johal, A., Thomson, R., Nicholl, J., Franklin, B., et al. (2008c). An epistemology of patient safety research: A framework for study design and interpretation. Part 3. End points and measurement. *Quality and Safety in Health Care*, 17(3), 170–177.

Brown, C.A. & Lilford, R.J. (2006). The stepped wedge trial design: A systematic review. *BMC Medical Research Methodology*, 6(1), 54.

Cardemil, C.V., Gilroy, K.E., Callaghan-Koru, J.A., Nsona, H., & Bryce, J. (2012). Comparison of methods for assessing quality of care for community case management of sick children. *American Journal of Tropical Medicine & Hygiene*, 87(5 Suppl), 127–136.

Chin-Quee, D., Bratt, J., Malkin, M., Nduna, M.M., Otterness, C., Jumbe, L., et al. (2013). Building on safety, feasibility, and acceptability: The impact and cost of community health worker provision of injectable contraception. *Global Health: Science & Practice*, 1(3), 316–327.

Cohen, J. (1988). *Statistical Power Analysis for the Behavioral Sciences*. Hillsdale, NJ, Lawrence Erlbaum.

Counihan, H., Harvey, S.A., Sekeseke-Chinyama, M., Hamainza, B., Banda, R., Malambo, T., et al. (2012). Community health workers use malaria rapid diagnostic tests (RDTs) safely and accurately: Results of a longitudinal study in Zambia. *American Journal of Tropical Medicine & Hygiene*, 87(1), 57–63.

Creswell, J.W. & Clark, V.L.P. (2017). *Designing and Conducting Mixed Methods Research* (Second Edition). Thousand Oaks, Sage publications.

Donner, A. & Klar, N. (2000). *Design and Analysis of Cluster Randomization Trials in Health Research*. London, Arnold.

Dunbar, E.L., Wroe, E.B., Nhlema, B., Kachimanga, C., Gupta, R., Taylor, C., et al. (2018). Evaluating the impact of a community health worker programme on non-communicable disease, malnutrition, tuberculosis, family planning and antenatal care in Neno, Malawi: Protocol for a stepped-wedge, cluster randomised controlled trial. *BMJ Open*, 8(7), e019473.

Gaziano, T.A., Abrahams-Gessel, S., Denman, C.A., Montano, C.M., Khanam, M., Puoane, T., et al. (2015). An assessment of community health workers' ability to screen for cardiovascular disease risk with a simple, non-invasive risk assessment instrument in Bangladesh,

Guatemala, Mexico, and South Africa: An observational study. *Lancet Global Health*, (9), e556–e563.

Gobezayehu, A.G., Mohammed, H., Dynes, M.M., Desta, B.F., Barry, D., Aklilu, Y., et al. (2014). Knowledge and skills retention among frontline health workers: Community maternal and newborn health training in rural Ethiopia. *Journal of Midwifery & Women's Health*, 59(s1), S21–S31.

Harvey, S.A., Jennings, L., Chinyama, M., Masaninga, F., Mulholland, K., & Bell, D.R. (2008). Improving community health worker use of malaria rapid diagnostic tests in Zambia: Package instructions, job aid and job aid-plus-training. *Malaria Journal*, 7(1), 160.

Hoffmann, T.C., Glasziou, P.P., Boutron, I., Milne, R., Perera, R., Moher, D., et al. (2014). Better reporting of interventions: Template for intervention description and replication (TIDieR) checklist and guide. *British Medical Journal*, 348, g1687.

Johnson, R.E., Grove, A.L., & Clarke, A. (2017). Pillar integration process: A joint display technique to integrate data in mixed methods research. *Journal of Mixed Methods Research*, doi. org/10.1177/1558689817743108.

Kirkpatrick, D. (1967). Evaluation of training. In R. Craig & I. Mittel (Eds). *Training and Development Handbook*. New York, McGraw Hill, pp. 87–112.

Kletter, M., Mendelez-Torres, G., Lilford, R., & Taylor, C. (2018). A library of logic models to explain how interventions to reduce diagnostic errors work. *Journal of Patient Safety*. doi: 10.1097/PTS.0000000000000459.

Kneale, D., Thomas, J., & Harris, K. (2015). Developing and optimising the use of logic models in systematic reviews: Exploring practice and good practice in the use of programme theory in reviews. *PLoS ONE*, 10(11), e0142187.

Leigh, A. (2018). *Randomistas: How Radical Researchers Are Changing Our World*. London, Yale University Press.

Lilford, R.J. & Jackson, J. (1995). Equipoise and the ethics of randomization. *Journal of the Royal Society of Medicine*, 88(10), 552–559.

Lopes, S.C., Cabral, A.J., & de Sousa, B. (2014). Community health workers: To train or to restrain? A longitudinal survey to assess the impact of training community health workers in the Bolama Region, Guinea-Bissau. *Human Resources for Health*, 12, 8.

McCambridge, J. (2015). From question-behaviour effects in trials to the social psychology of research participation. *Journal of Psychology & Health*, 3(1), 72–84.

Msisuka, C., Nozaki, I., Kakimoto, K., Seko, M., & Ulaya, M.M. (2011). An evaluation of a refresher training intervention for HIV lay counsellors in Chongwe District, Zambia. *Journal of Social Aspects of HIV/AIDS*, 8(4), 204–209.

O'Cathain, A., Murphy, E., & Nicholl, J. (2010). Three techniques for integrating data in mixed methods studies. *British Medical Journal*, 341, c4587.

O'Donovan, J., Kabali, K., Taylor, C., Chukhina, M., Kading, J.C., Fuld, J., et al. (2018). The use of low-cost Android tablets to train community health workers in Mukono, Uganda, in the recognition, treatment and prevention of pneumonia in children under five: A pilot randomised controlled trial. *Human Resources for Health*, 16, 49.

Olaniran, A., Smith, H., Unkels, R., Bar-Zeev, S., & van den Broek, N. (2017). Who is a community health worker? A systematic review of definitions. *Global Health Action*, 10(1), 1272223.

Plowright, A., Taylor, C., Davies, D., Sartori, J., Lewando Hundt, G., & Lilford, R. (2018). Formative evaluation of a training intervention for community health workers in South Africa: A before and after study. *PLoS ONE*, 13(9), e0202817.

Redick, C. & Dini, H. (2014). *The Current State of CHW Training Programs in sub-Saharan Africa and South Asia: What we know, what we don't know and what we need to do*. Available from: http://1millionhealthworkers.org/files/2013/01/1mCHW_mPowering_LitReview_ Formatted.compressed.pdf

Saravanan, S., Turrell, G., Johnson, H., Fraser, J., & Patterson, C.M. (2012). Re-examining authoritative knowledge in the design and content of a TBA training in India. *Midwifery*, 2(1), 120–130.

Shrivastava, S. & Shrivastava, P. (2012). Evaluation of trained Accredited Social Health Activist (ASHA) workers regarding their knowledge, attitude and practices about child health. *Rural Remote Health*, 1(4), 2099.

Solomon, R.L. (1949). An extension of control group design. *Psychological Bulletin*, 46(2), 137–150.

Surry, L.T., Torre, D., & Durning, S.J. (2017). Exploring examinee behaviours as validity evidence for multiple-choice question examinations. *Medical Education*, 51(10), 1075–1085.

Taljaard, M., Lilford, R., Girling, A., & Hemming, K. (2015). The stepped wedge cluster randomised trial: An opportunity to increase the quality of evaluations of service delivery and public policy interventions. *Trials*, 16(2), 1.

Taylor, C., Nhlema, B., Wroe, E., Aron, M., Makungwa, H., & Dunbar, E. (2018). Determining whether Community Health Workers are 'deployment ready' using standard setting. *Annals of Global Health*, 84(4), 630–639.

Uzochukwu, B., Onwujekwe, O., Ezeilo, E., Nwobi, E., & Ndu, A. (2008). Integrated management of childhood illness in Nigeria: Does short-term training of health workers improve their performance? *Journal of Public Health*, 122(4), 367–370.

Wass, V., Van der Vleuten, C., Shatzer, J., & Jones, R. (2001). Assessment of clinical competence. *Lancet*, 357(9260), 945–949.

11

Recognition, Mutual Respect, and Support

A Relational Approach to Training and Supervision in Community Health Work

Maureen Kelley and Nigel Fancourt

Introduction

Community health workers (CHWs) serve as an essential bridge between households, communities, and health facilities. They connect rural communities with health information and services and provide a sometimes underappreciated stopgap within struggling health systems, particularly in low resource settings in a world facing a predicted shortage of over 14 million health workers (WHO, 2018; Winters, O'Donovan & Geniets, 2018). As neighbours, family members, and friends of those in the communities served, CHWs have an intimate knowledge of lived health experiences in their own communities. They are typically relied upon as a means of translating and delivering community health interventions, but also offer valuable insights into understanding the priorities and needs of communities. Recognition of the importance of CHWs (Bhutta et al., 2010; Earth Institute, 2011; WHO, 2018) and pressure to address the predicted worldwide shortage of professional healthcare workers (Joint Learning Initiative, 2004) have fuelled recent government and private philanthropic efforts to scale up large CHW training programmes (Campbell et al., 2013; Cheney, 2018). As reliance on CHWs increases we have an opportunity and responsibility to critically reflect on the values and ethical commitments that have implicitly guided community health work and to consider what values ought to guide training and implementation strategies moving forward.

The ethical culture of a practice is in part shaped and reinforced by training and learning. In this chapter, we consider the values that have shaped professional and community views about the worth and role of CHWs and reflect on the residual impact on CHWs as learners. We argue for greater attention to the inherent worth of CHWs, recognition of their expertise and the value of their positionality in communities, both in their education and in practice. We consider the burdens of care shouldered by CHWs and the importance of educating CHWs to manage moral distress in

Maureen Kelley and Nigel Fancourt, *Recognition, Mutual Respect, and Support* In: *Training for Community Health*. Edited by: Anne Geniets, James O'Donovan, Laura Hakimi, and Niall Winters, Oxford University Press. © Oxford University Press 2021. DOI: 10.1093/oso/9780198866244.003.0011

their work by ensuring robust ethics planning and supervision. With the recent shift toward a model of shared decision-making and co-production of health in the global health agenda, respectful partnerships will be the cornerstone for successful community health programmes (Crisp & Chen, 2014). Yet, surprisingly little attention has been given to the role of relationships in training or to the particular ethical principles that support such working relationships. Throughout, we draw on work on the ethical character of relationships in workplace settings, and on learning how to collaborate between different types of expertise to guide training, supervision, and practice, with special attention to CHW programmes in the global south.

More than a 'Stopgap' Measure: Promoting the Lasting Value of Respectful Community Health Partnerships

Essential to any sustainable, effective collaboration is an attitude of mutual respect between partners and a sense of self-worth in respective roles. One of the sources of burnout and dissatisfaction for primary care providers in low and middle-income countries (LMICs) is lack of respect from health professionals and others who rely on CHWs in health delivery programmes (Jaskiewicz & Tulenko, 2012; Dugani et al., 2018). The causes of disrespectful treatment may be difficult to trace across diverse programmes, but possible factors include the hierarchical nature of health systems and lack of attention to this issue in health professional training and community health policy. Despite being recognized as a critical role in health delivery for more than four decades, CHWs have for a long time simply been considered part of a pragmatic agenda, as a bridge to essential health services where 'the alternative is no care at all' (Haines et al., 2007; Standing & Chowdhury, 2008). Recently, at the policy level there has been 'growing recognition' of the value of CHWs (WHO, 2018, p. 13), though also acknowledgment that 'support for CHWs and their integration into health systems and communities are uneven across and within countries' (p. 12). (See Panjabi et al. in Chapter 2 for further discussion.) Viewing the CHW role as merely pragmatic or non-ideal at the level of health systems or policy risks sending a message to government agencies, funders, and other organizations that CHW programmes are merely stopgap measures rather than long-term, essential roles in developing and developed health systems alike.

Equally importantly, a starting point of respect and recognition or one of expediency may influence interpersonal relationships between CHWs and health professionals, relationships which are vital to delivering improved care through community health system partnerships. Failing to attend to the 'practices of power' in implementation programmes, perpetuates inequalities across relationships that are central to the success of integrated community-based health programmes (Lehman & Gilson, 2013). The unintended consequence of serving as a perennial stopgap measure for chronic health systems shortcomings is that CHWs are not always given the recognition enjoyed by their professional counterparts (Cheney, 2018), often experiencing discrimination (Ajuebor et al., 2019). Unsurprisingly, they particularly value 'respectful collaboration and communication' (Scott et al., 2018).

Education and training can play into these structural inequalities and shape the culture of practice. Unlike health professionals, typically understood to be those completing three or more years of secondary education in the health sciences, and para-health professionals, those completing some post-secondary education, CHWs are typically lay health workers with no secondary education. Where health professionals are typically salaried and on contracts, in many countries CHWs work as volunteers or receive a small allowance; others are paid minimal wages. In this way, the financial value of the work is linked to the quality and quantity of education, creating an implicit hierarchy of healthcare employment. The education, training, and supervision of CHWs then reinforces that this is their place within the professional hierarchy, and the curriculum and pedagogy is decided accordingly. However, we are beginning to see a shift in practice. In many middle and high-income countries, such as the USA, South Africa, and India, there has been a move to certify, salary, and integrate CHWs within government health systems (Singh & Chokshi, 2013). Even in settings of extreme poverty, such as Haiti, organizations like Partners in Health have advocated for aligning CHW programmes with health systems and improving financing (Kim et al., 2013). Such efforts represent important models for shifting the professional culture and work environment for CHWs. Importantly, material and other forms of recognition better reflect CHWs' own sense of esteem and pride taken in the creativity and resourcefulness demonstrated in their daily work (Oliver et al., 2015).

Alongside the pragmatic agenda there has been renewed interest in the more idealistic origins of the primary healthcare movement sparked by Alma-Ata in 1978 a vision of CHWs as respected and valued agents of change from within communities (WHO, 1978; Standing & Chowdhury, 2008; Kane et al., 2016;). However, the educational implications of this vision have not been fully realized, partly because, since Alma-Ata, economic constraints and market-driven models of health delivery have increased pressure to deliver on the ideals of universal health access by cheap and cost-effective means (Winters et al., 2018). As such there is still a tendency to view CHWs as an extension of the health system rather than a catalyst for community empowerment, and the relational features of the work are overlooked (Werner, 1977; Haines et al., 2007; Glenton et al., 2010).

Respect is in many ways key here, and it includes both a general respect that is often demanded of everyone, akin to and arising out of a sense of solidarity, with the particular manifestations of respect one might show to certain categories of other people, such as a patient, a patient's relatives, community leaders, or other more qualified health professionals. Respect for the patient involves care, compassion and empathy, whereas respect for a malaria researcher involves politeness, trust, and attention. It is not a uniform duty, or rather must be enacted differently to different persons. The difficulty lies in judging the right form of respect to show and is linked to status, both for

CHWs in showing respect to various others, but also in having expectations about the kinds of respect that are owed to them, as a practice of power itself.

Rooted in a commitment to respect and solidarity, various programmes, such as the lady health worker initiative in Pakistan, have resisted the pragmatic paradigm of cost effectiveness by investing in greater training and support for CHWs (Rabbani et al., 2016). Increasingly, we are beginning to see an approach to CHWs that follows the principled commitments set out by Partners in Health, recognizing CHWs as: (1) professional members of care teams; (2) essential bridges between health systems and communities; and (3) as valued and critically important as health professionals in low resource settings (Palazuelos et al., 2018). This new model challenges the idea of CHW and paraprofessional care as second best and community-based healthcare as 'better than nothing' and rather returns to the idea of the community as a potentially powerful space for social justice in health. With an eye to developing a philosophy of training, this model offers a helpful starting point for considering how to operationalize respect for the worth and unique contributions of CHWs as agents of change in communities.

Educationally, there are three broad themes in considering the educational dimensions of CHWs. First, there is the question of how we conceive of the nature of the professionalism and especially the ethical decision-making of CHWs. Different professions call upon different commitments and values (impartiality in lawyers, fairness in teachers) and they may also have different ways of identifying and reconciling these commitments and values (MacIntyre, 1981; Applbaum, 1999; Hall, 2005). Given these values and commitments, we should then pay attention to when and how these should be learned. One might consider some values to be innate, or simply require them as pre-existing qualities of any potential CHW, so that there is no need to address them in training. Others might simply be considered to be only learned through experience, 'on the job'. Most will be learned or developed through education, but different models of education will be more or less effective at this. Finally, the relationship between professional ethics and educational ethics of any training will be important, not least because any educational programme is likely to have its own 'hidden curriculum' that is, over and above the formal curriculum, an implicit set of ideas and practices sending oblique and potentially counterproductive messages (Hafferty & Franks, 1994). For example, a programme for CHWs that was totally taught by healthcare professionals would send an implicit message about who is valued, and whose knowledge or expertise matters. We would therefore expect some congruence across health professional and CHW training.

Fostering Respect for CHW Contributions: Expanding the Boundaries of Expertise

Taking a relational approach to respectful partnership means fostering appreciation for the value of knowledge and expertise offered by CHWs through the approach and content of training. Central to this idea is recognition of CHWs as 'experience based experts'—where language, culture, social norms, and community trust are valued on par with medical and technological knowledge (Powell, 2006; Gilkey et al., 2011). In focused, technical interventions on constrained timelines, the learning content and preparation of CHWs may focus on building technical expertise but this content can nonetheless be delivered in ways that are mindful of what CHWs bring to the training. As trainers and teachers, this requires expanding the boundaries of what counts as expertise in learning contexts and greater appreciation of 'everyday understanding' (Collins & Evans, 2002). Explaining how a rapid test for malaria works with a group of CHWs might invite discussion about the best time of day to administer the test to allow families to attend to normal harvest times, or a discussion of how best to explain the test in the local language—both essential knowledge to implementing the rapid test successfully.

Since much of daily work of CHWs is emotional and social labour, our views of expertise need to expand to include these essential but often unrecognized skills. This work includes the difficult and sustained efforts of navigating power structures and social norms, building relationships and trust within the community and with representatives and outreach workers from the health system, government agencies, and NGOs (Maes & Kalofonos, 2013). With the majority of CHW positions filled by women (WHO, 2018), this shift in recognition of the value of emotional and social labour will require that we take a critical stance to entrenched gendered norms and attitudes about 'women's work' and its worth in the highly gendered political economy of global health (George, 2008; Maes et al., 2010; Kane et al., 2016).

These shifts in thinking can be fostered in the approach to CHWs as learners, but must also target approaches to training health professionals who interact with or supervise CHWs. Cultivating respect for local knowledge will shape how CHWs are treated in a particular learning moment and over time by health professionals and support staff. In hierarchical health and social systems where obtaining secondary and university education is a mark of social status, there are often substantial cultural and social barriers to cultivating mutual respect, as noted above. There can be strong norms of superiority for those who have gone away to university as well as deference on the part of some CHWs toward 'superiors' who serve as supervisors or links within hospitals and health systems. Gender may also play an role, for instance, having mostly male supervisors for mostly female CHWs may be inappropriate, reinforce gender barriers, and limit acceptability and effectiveness of supervision (WHO, 2018). Shifting culture will require changes in training content for health professionals, and novel approaches to interactive, bi-directional learning that engages the expertise of all partners in community health programmes and encourages active respect for what others in the partnership contribute to learning. A respectful, inclusive approach to training, will include encouraging health professionals to recognize their own sources of educational privilege and to see their degrees and certificates, not as a rite of passage to superior status, but as an opportunity to share this knowledge with others and to learn from others in the community.

Engaged and bi-directional modes of teaching will further cultivate self-worth and mutual respect for CHWs. Simple exposure to knowledge does not promote respectful engagement with active learners, no matter the educational background of participants. Participatory methods, such as photovoice (O'Donovan et al., 2019), are increasingly being acknowledged as tools for treating CHWs as active, curious learners with deep vested interest in directly contributing to health improvements in their communities. Such training has further potential to engage community members' pride in making an integral contribution to a public good (see Chapter 2).

Indeed, this is but one example of a wider demand for different disciplines to work together. Different forms of knowledge are increasingly divergent and specialized, as new fields and sub-fields emerge, and this is only possible though the creation of clear disciplinary and professional structures, with the concomitant epistemological and ethical standards: to be an oncologist is not to be a paediatrician, nor an occupational therapist. However, as a result, there are more calls for these specialisms to learn to collaborate and cooperate, to work on 'wicked problems' because their complexity makes them almost intractable (Ritchey, 2011). To address these issues, there are increasing demands for working together across disciplinary and professional divides, and for finding ways of thinking about how different professionals should work together.

In terms of CHWs' professional values, this means having confidence in their own professionalism as part of the shared solution to these issues, and therefore neither doubting their own professional standing when confronted by the professional hierarchies of medicine, nor denigrating the potential contributions of others, who may lack any formal education. Their position as mediators between, on one hand, patients and communities who have specific knowledge of contexts and conditions but lack medical expertise, and on the other, those with more institutionalized knowledge, which is more generalizable but potentially quasi-abstract in real world settings. This means valuing local knowledge and the 'experience-based expert', and getting beyond technological knowledge (Powell, 2006), in recognizing what counts as expertise (Collins & Evans, 2002).

This account of the relational ethics of CHWs has begun to show the complexity of their roles in balancing different demands and obligations. Key to this is recognizing that their education is not simply being 'given' technical information about procedures and treatments for essential and preventive health services but is about developing their agentic capacity through practical reasoning (Fulford et al., 2012). Indeed, they are required to combine this technical understanding and practical knowhow with an awareness of the underlying scientific and medical explanations, and with the complex relational issues outlined above, from dealing with patients and communities to implementing new system-level strategies at a local level.

There are clear implications for their education here, notably treating CHWs as agentic adult learners, for whom education and development will be ongoing. Indeed, they will also need to learn how to develop their own practice in the future, both as reflective individuals (Schön, 1983; Eraut, 1994), and also within professional groups, such as 'communities of practice' (Le May & Wenger, 2008), or 'relational expertise' (Edwards, 2010). Here, approaches that model or build on practice are valuable, through enquiry-led, problem-solving, developmental case studies that require agentic action, and thereby become educative, rather than simply demanding memorization and recall. Some examples would range from problem-based learning, particularly around increasingly complex case studies, in which a scenario can be presented simply and then adjusted and developed, to developing practice-based learning.

Beyond informing training with messages of mutual respect between health professionals and CHWs, other key features of CHW programmes and institutional design signal respect. Foremost is valuing the work and contributions through fair pay. Increasingly, fair compensation is expected and required in international guidance on CHW programmes and yet many programmes still involve volunteers or offer nominal pay for work (WHO, 2008; Maes et al., 2010; Olaniran et al., 2017; Palazuelos, 2018). While the desire to serve one's community by contributing to improvements in health is an important motivator for many CHWs, there is no strong evidence to support the view that fair compensation undermines this volunteer spirit for most. In cultural contexts where there are concerns expressed directly by the CHWs that wages may undermine a civic, religious, or cultural sense of duty, other modes of compensation can be negotiated with CHWs through prior engagement (Glenton et al., 2010). Non-monetary markers of recognition and fair commitment include investment in skills training that has value to a CHW outside a particular, narrow health intervention. For longer standing programmes this may include a pathway to professionalism, where feasible and desired by CHWs. Ethnographic research can contribute to our understanding of the range of expectations and motivations of CHWs, which include fair compensation, useful skills and employment opportunities, learning, meaningful relationships with those helped by their work, and altruistic goals, such as contributing the health of one's community, relieving suffering, or being of service in a religious or cultural sense (Kironde & Klaasen, 2002; Swidler & Watkins, 2009; Akintola, 2013; Maes & Kalofonos, 2013). Training programmes can be more responsive to context by engaging communities well before implementation and by building on other successful programmes in the region—both require sufficient financial support and timelines to accommodate planning, as well as cooperation across institutional boundaries to share information and lessons learned.

Moral Distress in the Face of Structural Needs: Ethics Training, Supervision, and Support

CHWs shoulder substantial responsibilities of care and in low resource settings face complex, unmet needs. Many such needs are due to structural determinants such as poverty, conflict, or geography. A common challenge faced by both health professionals and CHWs alike is the emotional distress of knowing what should be done (e.g. feeding one's family) but not being able to do what is morally right (the community is experiencing a drought and food insecurity). In the clinical context, rooted in nursing ethics, this phenomenon has become known as 'moral distress' (Campbell et al., 2016; Dudzinski, 2016). Because this emotional distress emanates from deeply felt obligations toward fellow human beings when face to face with suffering, it is especially strong on the front-lines of care—with nurses, social workers, aid workers, field researchers, and CHWs—and yet very little attention is given to equipping front-line caregivers to manage this distress. For CHWs who find the most meaning in helping fellow community members, being unable to help with serious economic and social needs is a source of stress and frustration (Maes, 2013). One of the most difficult features of moral distress in low resource settings is that one's sense of obligation to respond to complex health and social needs encountered in community work is deeply felt, while sustainable responses require structural, institutional, and political solutions that feel out of reach. Over time, chronic confrontation with complex, unmet needs can contribute to the sense of hopelessness and burnout (Zulu et al., 2014).

Recent research has developed effective tools for measuring moral distress in clinical settings and could be adapted to the community health worker context (Lamiani et al., 2017). However, we lack effective training models for equipping health professionals and CHWs to respond to and cope with moral distress. Innovation and development of ethics modules suited to community health work are needed. There has been interesting work in nursing on developing skills of resilience, or the capacity to reduce one's stress in morally challenging lines of work, such as intensive care units (Monteverde, 2016). Here, resilience is understood as a coping response to moral sources of stress, situations viewed as morally wrong, or in the face of moral dilemmas. What characterizes these situations is that no matter what one does, the need is not met, or the harm has merely been minimized, so coping involves recognition of the limits of what can be done, and doing one's best in such circumstances (Monteverde, 2016). A limitation to seeking solutions to moral distress through models of resilience is that it places the onus on the person experiencing distress to learn coping strategies as opposed to addressing the underlying causes of a morally harmful situation or injustice. Importantly, managers and health professionals face the same structural drivers of inequity and struggle to effect lasting change. A potential approach to training and preparation, drawing from experiences of front-line community researchers and community advisory boards, is to establish proactive plans to connect community members to available services and to identify tangible opportunities for collective advocacy across community and health professional networks. This requires robust, supportive supervision and familiarity with the local health and social systems (Madede et al., 2017).

Relational Agency and Empowerment of CHWs

The relational turn in clinical ethics followed important work in social science on the relational nature of agency and empowerment—namely, that meaningful accounts of a person's ability to act and engage in daily life should recognize that these are deeply influenced by and made possible by important relationships with others, including partners, family, friends, community members, and co-workers (Abrams, 1999; Archer & Maccarini, 2013). In ethics, important concepts, like autonomy and solidarity, have been reconsidered to acknowledge social influence and the value of relationships in determining right action and the scope of obligations to others (MacKenzie & Stoljar, 2000; Jennings, 2016).

Recognizing the value of relational clinical ethics presents a challenge to training and supervision, and in parallel, educational theories of work-based learning have had a relational turn, giving rise to new models of agentic learning in socially embedded contexts. One important theoretical contribution was Lave and Wenger's notion of 'situated learning', in which they pay attention to how collective knowledge develops through shared learning, and this has informed understandings of professional development across many disciplines and professions (Lave & Wenger, 1991; Le May & Wenger, 2009), though this work has been largely overlooked in CHW training (Winters et al., 2019). Others have highlighted how agentic and empowered professionals collaborate in the development of collective knowledge, for example Edwards (2010; 2017) has drawn on cultural-historical and activity theory (Daniels et al. 2010) to explore how individuals learn to work together, engaging with each other's expertise, through a developing 'relational agency' and a shared 'common knowledge'. And Nuttall (2017) has considered the implication of her work for learning within hospital hierarchies. These theories echo some of the findings of Vu Henry (Chapter 7), that simplistic models of learning are insufficient to account for the nuanced development of practices. Pedagogically, as noted above, the use of case studies as a form of problem-based learning has proved invaluable in developing inter-professional practices (e.g. Flaherty et al., 2003), as well as the direct involvement of patients (Wykurz & Kelly, 2002; Towle, 2007).

Exciting, recent work applies insights from relational ethics to CHWs' empowerment. Using Lee and Koh's analytic framework for empowerment, Kane et al. conducted a multi-country comparative study of CHW programmes in six LMICs and assessed CHW empowerment on four dimensions: meaningfulness, competence, self-determination, and impact (Kane et al., 2016). These case studies illustrate how organizational arrangements in LMIC community health programmes either promote or frustrate CHW empowerment along these dimensions. Reflecting on work in organizational studies they consider the potential tension between supervision and digital communication technology as a model of control and empowerment as a degree of independent self-determination (Hardy & O'Sullivan, 1998; Maynard et al., 2012). Following earlier work in psychology they argue that for CHWs in LMICs, 'there is nothing in the psychological definition of empowerment that requires the increase of power of one group to decrease the power of another group; power does not have to be seen as a zero-sum commodity, but can be a 'win-win' situation' (Swift & Levin, 1987; Kane et al., 2016). Relational agency gives greater scope and flexibility to guide this balancing act and encourages an approach to supervision which is supportive rather than controlling, but at the same time providing critical guidance when CHWs encounter situations that fall outside their clinical abilities (WHO, 2008). However, one of the challenges in striking this balance within working relationships is that shifting from a mode of empowerment to one of more authoritative supervision can be jarring if not done delicately. More engaged, long-term supervision can be both respectful and encouraging, and yet setting important boundaries when task shifting would raise concerns about clinical errors, but this is a skillset requiring careful training and experience for supervisors and CHWs in cultural contexts where authority and hierarchy sometimes take precedence over finding meaning in empowered work. One promising approach in training is to emphasize the non-clinical skills and contributions of CHWs during such boundary-setting (Naimoli et al., 2015).

Fairness and Inclusion

In addition to respect, another vital principle essential to ethically grounded CHW training is that of fairness—treating others with equal moral consideration within institutions and practices, and being mindful of patterns of discrimination that may need to be corrected to improve equity of representation. Grounded in the recognition of the equal worth of individuals, and like respect, fairness in a programme or practice is an ethical consequence of numerous norms, decisions, and moral attitudes toward one another. Indeed, fairness is entwined with respect, in that both require differential treatments of different people (Rawls, 2001). It means not unfairly favouring some in the community more than others, or prioritizing those who are in greatest need and most able to benefit from interventions, and recognizing that CHWs should be fair is implicitly to recognize that they have power to administer it, particularly in the distribution of and access to medical and health provision (Rawls, 2001). For example, CHWs may often find themselves in a position where they must decide who gets treatment access to care, or, 'Is the new clinic to be built in village A or village B?' Where principles of fairness guide us to give priority or greater consideration to those who are worst off in a community or society, CHWs may be in a position to ensure that a community health programme is designed optimally to give fair opportunity to all, not only those in a superior social or economic position (Rawls, 2001; Winters et al., 2020). Believing that the system should be fair means recognizing that it sometimes is not, either in terms of treatment (hence the need for advocacy, noted below) or in terms of the organizational hierarchies at stake. If the CHWs have some power, there are others within the wider medical community who have more. Finally, fairness also means not behaving selfishly or using the role for personal gain, as part of their professional responsibility, as outlined above. CHWs must judge themselves by the same standards and provide the same level of medical or healthcare to others as to themselves, their family, or those in power. Within an education programme, fairness needs to be both an explicit part of the curriculum, as an underpinning principle, but also inherently embedded within the educational processes, such as pedagogy and assessment (Winters et al., 2020).

Solidarity and Shared Advocacy

It is precisely in contexts of systematic and historical inequity where appeals to fairness and respect are not always enough to effect change at a programmatic level. As Benatar (2003), Harmon (2006), and Farmer et al. (2006) have independently argued, global health discourse has often overlooked the moral and politically transformative power of solidarity. Reconnecting with traditions of solidarity in community health calls on health workers at all levels and skill sets to recognize that we are in a shared struggle for a common purpose, that finding sustainable, more equitable solutions to complex structural problems will require structural, collective interventions. Jennings explains how we can reinvigorate public health ethics by paying attention not only to 'architectonic' ethical theorizing, at the level of principles, but also to 'relational' theorizing, with a combined appeal to solidarity and care ethics:

> Solidarity is characterized as affirming the moral standing of others and their membership in a community of equal dignity and respect. Care is characterized as paying attention to the moral (and mortal) being of others and their needs, suffering, and vulnerability. The wager of relational theorizing in health care and public health is that substantive ethical visions of solidarity and care will provide support for more just and egalitarian health care and public health policies.
>
> (Jennings, 2019, p. 4)

By recognizing our starting point in an interdependent world and reconnecting with the spirit of community spaces as a powerful place for change, community health programmes can be treated as part of the broader web of geographical and professional communities, across which both health information and practical strategies of social change have the potential to be shared more widely and more quickly than ever before (Frenk et al., 2010).

Building upon a shared responsibility is the obligation that flows from CHWs' solidarity with patients and communities to use their role as professional to speak out on behalf of patients and in setting community health priorities (Hoedemaekers & Dekkers, 2003). Thus, their responsibility is not simply to treat, as outlined above, but also to express, argue, and request—and perhaps complain and demand—on behalf of those needing care. This particularly applies to those who find the medical system hard to navigate for whatever reason—disability, poverty, age, gender, language, and perhaps prejudice. It is linked to fairness and inclusion. Clearly, it is one thing to expect a CHW to engage in advocacy, and another to expect a student to do so, but it should still be addressed in teaching or through practical experience. We, of course, do not envisage advocacy training as student lawyers would learn it, through moots and debates. Instead, it is through smaller encounters and raising awareness, encouraging active reflection on shared experience in training, and demonstrating a degree of self-worth and even courage in some situations. Here simulation-based approaches could be used, for instance asking CHWs to design a poster for a community on the treatment of disabled members of the community.

Ethical Principles to Guide a Relational Pedagogy

As we have shown, many of the challenges and perceptions discussed so far are relational and ethical in nature. Relational work requires skills in relationship-building and fostering the relational agency of CHWs through engaged supervision. As such, innovative training programmes for CHWs, health professionals, and supervisors could be improved by paying more explicit attention to building capacity in relational ethics. Emerging from clinical ethics in nursing and linked to feminist traditions in care ethics, relational ethics situates moral decision-making, actions, and obligations within relationship (Noddings, 1984; MacDonald, 2007; Gilligan, 2008; Gergen, 2009; Baylis et al., 2008; Held, 2005). As MacDonald has argued, practical ethics teaching following this tradition is concerned with more than teaching students to problem-solve in the face of ethical dilemmas, it is about developing the skills for living and working together. It is also highly sensitive to the context in which those relationships can be fostered and sustained. To this end she offers a pedagogical model based on four core principles: mutual respect, relational engagement, bringing knowledge to life, and creating environment, to better support nurses within roles of moral responsibility and advocacy (MacDonald, 2007). Building on these principles in the context of community health practice and incorporating more explicitly the values we have defended here, we have a useful framework to inform teaching and training for CHWs and health professionals engaged in supervision and support for CHW programmes. We illustrate how each principle can be grounded in professional commitments and inform innovative teaching methodologies and training content (see Table 11.1).

Clearly, the use of these strategies, and indeed the underpinning pedagogical assumptions will raise issues for the design of any assessment criteria, such as standards or competencies. These alignment issues are too complex to address in full, but might be met by the use of portfolios, reflective logs, or observation by experts. Put simply, assessment will also need rethinking. The hope is that by putting the values front and centre we can prompt meaningful consideration of practical ethics considerations as well as dialogue around the deeper systemic injustices that give rise to the desperate need for CHWs as a recognized and valued part of extended health systems.

Table 11.1 Putting ethical principles to work in CHW and health professional training programmes in LMICs

Ethical values and principles	Shared commitment	Practical illustration
Mutual respect and recognition	*We will demonstrate respect for patients, community members, and co-workers, acknowledging the values, choices, and knowledge they bring to the situation.*	A teaching session in rural Kenya begins with an interactive session of imaginative role reversal where CHWs and health professionals step inside each other's roles to appreciate challenges and mutual expertise.
Shared decision-making and solidarity	*We recognize that to achieve improved health for all requires our joint efforts across communities and health systems—we all have the same goal—improved health and a better life for our families and communities.*	After several emotionally challenging cases of domestic violence in their communities, CHWs, health professionals, and community leaders in South Africa convene a workshop with participatory theatre to bring violence in the home out into the open, exploring violence as a common challenge for them.
Relational agency and empowerment	*We are committed to offering the knowledge and support needed for patients, community members and co-workers to engage actively in their health and work.*	In interactive session with new CHWs asks them to solve a complex problem together, through case studies. The dialogue requires them to support and be supported by each other, and a debrief prompts participants to reflect on other ways of empowering each other by sharing knowledge.
Fairness and inclusion	*We are committed to fairness in treatment and support for all patients and co-workers, regardless of gender, ethnicity, disability, or socioeconomic background.*	Through a case study in which the vaccinations are not given fairly, favouring community leaders' extended families. CHWs are asked to consider how they should and would deliver the programme.
Shared advocacy	*We have a shared commitment to advocate for those in need of better health services and to connect patients to existing services where feasible.*	A new CHW programme decides to set aside time for supervisors, CHWs, and mothers to proactively develop an advocacy plan to address expected, urgent needs related to the new antenatal health programme.

Conclusion

It is over a decade on from the Lancet commission on Education of Health Professionals, which called for a transformation of health education to respond to increasing global interdependency, including new technologies, information networks, professional migration, and financing across borders (Frenk et al., 2010). As the global health community, development organizations, and governments set out aspirational targets for equity in health, development, and well-being for a global population through collective commitments like the Sustainable Development Goals, community health programmes need to be recognized as foundational to success (United Nations, 2015). We have reflected on how such commitments to relational ethics and social justice inform CHW and health professional training. Without this admittedly aspirational, shared commitment, there is a tendency for well-meaning, pragmatic efforts and programmes to devolve into siloed agendas with CHWs feeling disconnected and powerless to effect change on their own. We have argued for a shift in policy discourse and training philosophy that gives greater attention to building relationships and support to foster successful, sustainable community health programmes in an increasingly interdependent world.

References

Abrams, K. (1999). From autonomy to agency: Feminist perspectives on self-direction. *Hofstra Law Review*, 805(2), 243–258.

Ajuebor, O., Cometto, G., Boniol, M., & Akl, E. (2019). Stakeholders' perceptions of policy options to support the integration of community health workers in health systems. *Human Resources for Health*, 17(13).

Akintola, O., Hlengwa, M., & Dageid, W. (2013). Perceived stress and burnout among volunteer caregivers working in AIDS care in South Africa. *Journal of Advanced Nursing*, 69(12), 2738–2749.

Applbaum A. (1999). *Ethics for Adversaries: The Morality of Roles in Public and Professional Life*. Princeton, Princeton University Press.

Archer M.S. & Maccarini, A. (Eds) (2013). *Engaging with the World: Agency, Institutions, Historical Formations*. New York, Routledge.

Baylis, F., Kenny, N.P., & Sherwin, S. (2008). A relational account of public health ethics. *Public Health Ethics*, 1(3), 196–209.

Benatar, S.R., Daar, A.S., & Singer, P.A. (2003). Global health ethics: The rationale for mutual caring. *International Affairs*, 107–138.

Bhutta, Z.A., Lassi, Z.S., Pariyo, G., & Huicho, L. (2010). *Global Experience of Community Health Workers for Delivery of Health-Related Millennium Development Goals: A Systematic Review, Country Case Studies, and Recommendations for Integration into National Health Systems*. Geneva, World Health Organization.

Campbell, J. (2013). Towards universal health coverage: A health workforce fit for purpose and practice. *Bulletin of World Health Organization*, 91, 886–887.

Campbell, S., Ulrich, C.M., & Grady C. (2016). A broader understanding of moral distress. *American Journal of Bioethics*, 16(12), 2–9.

Cheney, C. (2018). New initiative leverages technology and philanthropy to reinvent community health care. Available from: http://devex.com/news/new-initiative-leverages-techonology-and-philanthropy-to-reinvent-community-health-care-91878

Collins, H.M. & Evans, R. (2002). The third wave of science studies: Studies of expertise and experience. *Social Studies of Science*, 32, 235–296.

Crisp, N. & Chen, L. (2014). Global supply of health professionals. *The New England Journal of Medicine*, 370(23), 2247–2248. doi:10.1056/NEJMc1404326. PMID: 24897096.

Daniels, H., Edwards, A., Engerström, Y., Gallagher, T., & Ludvigsen, S. (Eds) (2010). *Activity Theory in Practice: Promoting Learning Across Boundaries and Agencies*. London, Routledge.

Dudzinski, D.M. (2016). Navigating moral distress using the moral distress map. *Journal of Medical Ethics*, 42(5), 321–324.

Dugani S., Afari, H., Hirschhorn, L., Ratcliffe, H., Veillard, J., Martin, G., et al. (2018). Prevalence and factors associated with burnout among frontline primary health care providers in low- and middle-income countries: A systematic review. *Gates Open Research*, 11(2), 4.

Earth Institute (2011). *One Million Community Health Workers: Technical Taskforce Report, Earth Institute*. Available from: http://www.millenniumvillages.org/uploads/ReportPaper/1mCHW_TechnicalTaskForceReport.pdf

Edwards, A. (2010). *Being an Expert Professional Practitioner: The Relational Turn in Expertise*. Berlin, Springer.

Edwards, A. (Ed.) (2017). *Working Relationally in and Across Practices: A Cultural-historical Approach to Collaboration*. Cambridge, Cambridge University Press.

Eraut, M. (1994). *Developing Professional Knowledge and Competence*. London, Falmer Press.

Farmer, P. Nizeye, B., Stulac, S., & Keshavjee, S. (2006). Structural violence and clinical medicine. *PLoS Medicine*, 3(10), 1686–1691.

Flaherty, E., Hyer, K., Kane, R., Wilson, N., Whitelaw, N., & Fulmer T. (2003). Using case studies to evaluate students' ability to develop a geriatric interdisciplinary care plan. *Gerontology & Geriatrics Education*, 24(2), 63–74.

Frenk, J., Chen, L., Bhutt, Z.A., Cohen, J., Crisp, N., Evans, T., et al. (2010). Health professional for a new century: Transforming education to strengthen health systems in an interdependent world. *Lancet*, 376, 1923–1958.

Fulford, K.W., Peile, E., & Carroll, H. (2012). *Essential Values-based Practice: Clinical Stories Linking Science with People*. Cambridge, Cambridge University Press.

George, A. (2008). Nurses, community health workers, and home carers: Gendered human resources compensating for skewed health systems. *Global Public Health*, 3(S1), 75–89.

Gergen, K.J. (2009). *Relational Being: Beyond Self and Community*. New York, NY, Oxford University Press.

Gilkey, M., Cochran Garci, C., & Rush, C. (2011). Professionalization and the experience-based expert: Strengthening partnerships between health educators and community health workers. *Health Promotion Practice*, 12(2), 178–182.

Gilligan, C. (2008). Moral orientation and moral development. In: A. Bailey & C.J. Cuomo (Eds). *The Feminist Philosophy Reader*. Boston, McGraw-Hill, pp. 467–477.

Glenton, C., Scheel, I.B., Pradhan, S., Lewin, S., Hodgins, S., & Shrestha, V. (2010). The female community health volunteer programme in Nepal: Decision makers' perceptions of volunteerism, payment and other incentives. *Social Science & Medicine*, 70(12), 1920–1927.

Hafferty, F.W. & Franks, R. (1994). The hidden curriculum, ethics teaching, and the structure of medical education. *Academic Medicine: Journal of the Association of American Medical Colleges*, 69(11), 861–871.

Haines, A., Sanders, A., Lehmann, U., Rowe, A.K., Lawn, J.E., Jan, S., et al. (2007). Achieving child survival goals: Potential contribution of community health workers. *Lancet*, 369(9579), 2121–2131.

Hall, P. (2005). Interprofessional teamwork: Professional cultures as barriers. *Journal of Interprofessional Care*, 19(1), 188–196.

Hardy, C. & Leiba-O'Sullivan, S. (1998). The power behind empowerment: Implications for research and practice. *Human Relations*, 51(4), 451–483.

Harmon, S.H.E. (2006). Solidarity: A (new) ethic for global health policy. *Health Care Analysis*, 14(4), 215–236.

Held, V. (2005). *The Ethics of Care: Personal, Political and Global*. New York, NY: Oxford University Press.

Hoedemaekers, R. & Dekkers, W. (2003). Justice and solidarity in priority setting in health care. *Health Care Analysis*, 11(4), 325–343.

Jaskiewicz, W. & Tulenko, K. (2012). Increasing community health worker productivity and effectiveness: A review of the influence of the work environment. *Human Resources for Health*, 10, 38.

Jennings, B. (2016). Reconceptualizing autonomy: The relational turn in bioethics. *Hastings Center Report*, 46(3), 11–16.

Jennings, B. (2019). Relational ethics for public health: Interpreting solidarity and care. *Health Care Analysis*, 27(1), 4–12.

Joint Learning Initiative (2004). *Human Resources for Health—Overcoming the Crisis*. Cambridge: Joint Learning Initiative. Available from: www.who.int/hrh/documents/JLi_hrh_report.pdf

Kane, S., Kok, M., Ormel, H., Otiso, L., Sidat, M., Namakhoma, I., et al. (2016). Limits and opportunities to community health worker empowerment: A multi-country comparative study. *Social Science and Medicine*, 164, 27–34.

Kim, J.Y., Porter, M., Rhatigan, J., Weintraub, R., Basilico, M., van der Hoof Holstein, C., et al. (2013). Scaling up effective delivery models worldwide. In: P. Farmer, J. Yong Kim, A. Kleinman, & M. Basilico (Eds). *Reimagining Global Health*. Berkeley, UC Press, pp. 184–211.

Kironde, S. & Klaasen, S. (2002). What motivates lay volunteers in high burden but resource-limited tuberculosis control programmes? Perceptions from the Northern Cape province, South Africa. *International Journal of Tuberculosis & Lung Disease*, 6(2), 104–110.

Lamiani, G., Setti, I., Barlascini, L., Vegni, E., & Argentero, P. (2017). Measuring moral distress among critical care clinicians: Validation and psychometric properties of the Italian moral distress scale-revised. *Critical Care Medicine*, 45(3), 430–437.

Lave, J. & Wenger, E. (1991). *Situated Learning: Legitimate Peripheral Participation*. Cambridge, Cambridge University Press.

Lehmann, U. & Gilson, L. (2013). Actor interfaces and practices of power in a community health worker programme: A South African study of unintended policy outcomes. *Health Policy and Planning*, 28(4), 358–366.

Le May, A. & Wenger, E. (2008). *Communities of Practice in Health and Social Care*. London, Wiley-Blackwell.

MacDonald, H. (2007). Relational ethics and advocacy in nursing: Literature review. *Journal of Advanced Nursing*, 57(2), 119–126.

MacIntyre, A. (1981). *After Virtue: A Study In Moral Theory*. Chicago, University of Notre Dame Press.

Mackenzie, C. & Stoljar, N. (Eds) (2000). *Relational Autonomy Feminist Perspectives on Autonomy, Agency and the Social Self*. New York, Oxford University Press.

Madede, T., Sidat, M., McAuliffe, E., Patricio, S.R., Uduma, O., Galligan, M., et al. (2017). The impact of a supportive supervision intervention on health workers in Niassa, Mozambique: A cluster-controlled trial. *Human Resources for Health*, 15(1), 58.

Maes, K.C., Kohrt, B.A. & Closser, S. (2010). Culture, status and context in community health worker pay: Pitfalls and opportunities for policy research. *Social Science & Medicine*, 71, 1375–1378.

Maes, K. & Kalofonos, I. (2013). Becoming and remaining community health workers: Perspectives from Ethiopia and Mozambique. *Social Science & Medicine*, 87, 52–59.

Maynard, M., Gilson, L., & Mathieu, J. (2012). Empowerment—Fad or Fab? A multilevel review of the past two decades of research. *Journal of Management*, 38(4), 1231–1281.

Monteverde, S. (2016). Caring for tomorrow's workforce: Moral resilience and healthcare ethics education. *Nursing Ethics*, 23(1), 104–116.

Naimoli, J., Perry, H., Townsend, J., Frymus, D., & McCaffery, J. (2015). Strategic partnering to improve community health worker programming and performance: Features of a community-health system integrated approach. *Human Resources for Health*, 13(46), 1–13.

Noddings, N. (1984). *Caring: A Feminine Approach to Ethics and Moral Education*. Berkeley, University of California Press.

Nuttall J. (2017). Learning and deploying relational agency in the negotiation of interprofessional hierarchies in a UK Hospital. In: A. Edwards (Ed.). *Working Relationally in and Across Practices: A Cultural-historical Approach to Collaboration*. Cambridge, Cambridge University Press, pp. 43–57.

O'Donovan, J., Hamala, R., Namanda, A.S., Musoke, D., Ssemugabo, C., & Winters, N. (2019). We are the people whose opinions don't matter. A photovoice study exploring challenges faced by community health workers in Uganda. *Global Public Health*, 15(3), 384–401.

Olaniran, A., Smith, H., Unkels, R., Bar-Zeev, S., & van den Broek, N. (2017). Who is a community health worker?—A systematic review of definitions. *Global Health Action*, 10(1), 1272223.

Oliver, M., Geniets, A., Winters, N., Rega, I., & Mbae, S.M. (2015). What do community health workers have to say about their work, and how can this inform improved programme design? A case study with CHWs within Kenya. *Global Health Action*, 8, 27168.

Palazuelos, D., Farmer, P., & Mukherjee, J. (2018). Community health and equity of outcomes: The Partners in Health experience. *Lancet*, 6(5), e491–e493.

Powell, M. (2006). Which knowledge? Whose reality? An overview of knowledge used in the development sector. *Development in Practice*, 16(6), 518–532.

Rabbani, F.L., Shipton, W., Aftab, W., Sangrasi, K., Perveen, S., & Zahidie, A. (2016). Inspiring health worker motivation with supportive supervision: A survey of lady health supervisor motivating factors in rural Pakistan. *BMC Health Services Research*, 16(1), 397.

Rawls J. (2001). *Justice as Fairness: A Restatement*. Cambridge, Harvard University Press.

Ritchey, T. (2011). *Wicked Problems—Social Messes: Decision Support Modelling with Morphological Analysis*. Berlin, Springer.

Schön, D. (1983). *The Reflective Practitioner: How Professionals Think in Action*. London, Temple Smith.

Scott, K., Beckham, S.W., Gross, M., Pariyo, G., Rao. K., Cometto, G., & Perry, H. (2018). What do we know about community-based health worker programs? A systematic review of existing reviews on community health workers. *Human Resources for Health*, 16, 39.

Singh, P. & Chokshi, D.A. (2013). Community health workers—a local solution to a global problem. *New England Journal of Medicine*, 369(10), 894–896.

Standing, H. & Chowdhury A.M. (2008). Producing effective knowledge agents in a pluralistic environment: What future for community health workers? *Social Science and Medicine*, 66(10), 2096–2107.

Swidler, A. & Watkins, S.C. (2009). 'Teach a Man to Fish': The doctrine of sustainability and its effects on three strata of Malawian society. *World Development*, 37(7), 1182–1196.

Swift, C. & Levin, G. (1987). Empowerment: An emerging mental health technology. *The Journal of Primary Prevention*, 8(1–2), 71–94.

Towle, A. (2007). Involving patients in the education of health care professionals. *Journal of Health Services Research & Policy*, 12(1), 1–2.

United Nations General Assembly (2015). Sustainable Development Goals: 17 Goals to transform our world. Available from https://www.un.org/sustainabledevelopment/sustainable-development-goals/ [Accessed 18 February 2021].

Werner, D. (1977). The village health worker: Lackey or liberator? Proceedings of International Hospital Federation Congress 22–27 May 1977. Available from: http://www.healthwrights.org/content/articles/lackey_or_liberator.htm

Winters, N., O'Donovan, J., & Geniets, A. (2018). A new era for community health in countries of low and middle income. *Lancet*, 6(May), e489.

Winters, N., Langer, L., Nduku, P., Robson, J., O'Donovan, J., Maulik, P., et al. (2019). Using mobile technologies to support the training of community health workers in low-income and middle-income countries: Mapping the evidence. *BMJ Global Health*, 4(4), e001421.

Winters N, Venkatapuram, S., Geniets, A., & Wynne-Bannister, E. (2020). Prioritarian principles for digital health in low resource settings. *Journal of Medical Ethics*, doi:10.1136/medethics-2019-105468.

World Health Organization (1978). Declaration of Alma-Ata 1978. International conference of primary health care. Alma-Ata: USSR, 6–12 September 1978.

World Health Organization (2008). *Task Shifting: Rational Redistribution of Tasks Among Health Workforce Teams*. Geneva, World Health Organization.

World Health Organization (2018). *WHO Guideline on Health Policy and System Support to Optimize Community Health Worker Programmes*. Geneva, World Health Organization.

Wykurz, G. & Kelly, D. (2002). Developing the role of patients as teachers: Literature review. *BMJ (Clinical research ed.)*, 32 (7368), 818–821.

Zulu, J.M., Kinsman, J., Michelo, C., &. Hurtig, A.K. (2014). Hope and despair: Community health assistants' experiences of working in a rural district in Zambia. *Human Resources for Health*, 1478–4491, 12–30.

12
Conclusion

Towards a Pedagogy for Community Health Workers?

Laura Hakimi, Anne Geniets, James O'Donovan, and Niall Winters

Introduction

The Covid-19 pandemic took a grim hold across nations, putting enormous strain on even the most sophisticated, well-resourced health systems. The outbreak has served to lay bare the disparity between the world's health systems, in terms of their capacity, response strategies, and resources. It has exposed the health equity gaps in society within and between countries, and the resulting differences in health treatment, prophylaxis (due to a lack of vaccine equity between and within countries, with LMICs being disproportionately affected), and consequently, in many cases, health outcomes, that are due to socio-economic differences.

In previous disease outbreaks, the expansion of healthcare teams through CHWs has proven to be fundamental to an effective response. During the Ebola outbreak in the Democratic Republic of Congo (DRC) and West Africa, nations including Liberia, Sierra Leone, Guinea, Nigeria, and the DRC rapidly hired, trained, and equipped thousands of CHWs from communities affected by, or at risk from, the outbreak. As part of interdisciplinary teams of nurses, doctors, and other health workers, CHWs played a vital role in reducing transmission through promoting social distancing and contact tracing, detecting and referring individuals with suspected Ebola for testing, and encouraging Ebola patients to seek care early (see, e.g. Vandi et al., 2017; Heymann et al., 2015).

In this way, CHWs have been shown to be uniquely positioned to promote healthy household practices and appropriate healthcare-seeking behaviours, and to make an important contribution to controlling outbreaks by engaging and building trust within communities (Bhutta et al., 2010). With access to appropriate training, supervision, and support, CHWs can play a key role in community-based public health programmes, taking on the roles of health educators, making use of existing local social networks to create 'bonds of trust' between communities and health systems, and encouraging community members to access the nearest health services in times of need (Perry et al., 2016, p. 522). Such attributes are crucial in infectious disease outbreaks, where the 'the ability [of CHWs] to respond quickly... is likely to reduce

Laura Hakimi, Anne Geniets, James O'Donovan, and Niall Winters, *Conclusion* In: *Training for Community Health*. Edited by: Anne Geniets, James O'Donovan, Laura Hakimi, and Niall Winters, Oxford University Press. © Oxford University Press 2021. DOI: 10.1093/oso/9780198866244.003.0012

the risk of widespread infection' (ibid). In this way, CHWs are uniquely positioned to employ outreach, education, and community engagement strategies that can help to contain or, indeed, prevent outbreaks of disease. There is also evidence to suggest that deploying community health workers can contribute to the strengthening and rebuilding of health systems following health crises (Perry et al., 2014; 2016). At the same time, the Covid-19 pandemic has made apparent the global lack of good quality evidence and the need to train CHWs in collecting data in low and middle-income countries (LMICs). It has further highlighted the need for better global health information systems, which should integrate community, hospital, and government data and enable sharing for diagnoses, imaging, and lab results. The appropriate use of technology will be key to these efforts.

Health crises such as the Ebola epidemic and the Covid-19 pandemic have accentuated the importance of effective training, supervision, and support for CHWs, in a way that is pedagogically effective and adaptable to meet changing demands of health systems and the communities they serve. In this book we have outlined a number of approaches to train a CHW workforce, which are equitable and empowering, flexible and adaptable, and can continue to address health equity gaps and to support efforts to tackle health crises.

Some important themes cut across the book's varied and interdisciplinary chapters: the need for greater respect, value, and recognition of CHWs' unique contribution to health provision, including their community knowledge and experience; the need for greater attention to pedagogy in CHW training and supervision, particularly when using technology; the need for better use of research evidence to inform training programmes; and the use of participatory approaches for empowering and ethically appropriate training and supervision. We draw on our case studies to illustrate the ways in which these themes have been put into practice and point to some positive and exciting ways forward.

Value, Empowerment, and Professionalization

Many of the contributors to this book have emphasized the importance of respect for and value of CHWs. Rather than solely administrators of medical interventions, authors have been quick to articulate the important holistic, community based, and socially orientated role of CHWs. Rather than an 'extension' of the health system, CHWs should be positioned as an integral part of it, and, indeed, as a 'catalyst' for community empowerment, or agents of social change. Rather than a 'low-cost solution' to a shortage of health workers, there are 'significant opportunities to leverage their unique skills, address disparities and inequities in care and improve health outcomes' (Chapter 3). Furthermore, this book has discussed at length the digital empowerment of CHWs and recognized the importance of their role, for example in affecting treatment cycles and the evolution of frontline practice, for example to collect health metrics. In this way, this book has argued that CHWs may be placed at the very forefront of detection, public health interventions, and disease monitoring. Schaaf et al. (2018) suggest that a CHW's social position and professional role influence how they are treated and trusted by the health sector and by community members, as well as when, where, and how they can exercise agency and promote accountability. It is thus crucial to foster an appreciation for the value of their knowledge and expertise, and this should be reflected in the content, format, and pedagogical approach of their training.

However, to date, the training of CHWs has often overlooked the individual learning and empowerment of CHWs as health practitioners in favour of training approaches that are task- and process-focused leaving little room for the empowerment, growth, and development of CHWs (Winters et al., 2019; see also Chapter 9). Subsequently, training has failed to acknowledge and address the need to facilitate empowered and autonomous learners (Chapter 4). As made clear in Chapter 11, there is a danger that training and supervision of CHWs can serve to inadvertently reinforce structural inequalities.

Efforts to foster more respectful, empowering training opportunities must not be thought of in isolation from the broader professional experiences of CHWs. In Chapter 3 Palazuelos and Gadi argue that the empowerment of CHWs means providing them with all the elements necessary to work effectively (i.e. fair compensation for their time, other financial protections, robust training, and appropriate supervision and mentorship, so that they perform their tasks with excellence and fidelity). Yet, CHWs experience a variety of different circumstances in terms of job title, pay, social position, reporting structure, etc. There have been calls for the professionalization of the career path so that CHWs can be sure of a more equitable, consistent, accredited experience, as well as a sense of progression, recognition, and empowerment over the course of a CHW's working life. This reflects, within the institutional framework of a national or local health system, a more concrete mark of respect, and the value of CHW's role and expertise. In any career path, part of the process of professionalization is pedagogically sound training.

Embedding Learning Theory in Training and Supervision

Never has it been more important that training and supervision is pedagogically sound and effective at supporting the development of CHWs. Our chapter authors have argued strongly and consistently for greater attention to pedagogy in the design of CHW training and supervision. In Chapter 7 Vu Henry argues for not only an increased reflection on what it means to 'learn' when both phones and CHWs are mobile, but also addressing the implications this has for CHW training. More pragmatically speaking, there has been a shift beyond information dissemination to a more context-led, participatory approach. As Nagraj suggests in Chapter 6, the most important first step in designing a training and supervision intervention is to understand the needs of the learners and marry these with the needs and capacities of the teachers and the health system. With this in mind, Muso (see case study in appendix 3) co-creates training content with the CHW recipients. Much of Muso's activity comes from feedback from several generations of CHW cohorts. This organization recommends using CHW data to identify systemic practice issues and be prepared to use those lessons to adjust training approaches accordingly.

This picture is further complicated by the incorporation of technologies in any training or supervision programme. Technology-enhanced learning is a method of teaching delivery which may offer more flexibility to learners and teachers, particularly those working in environments where there are workforce constraints. In the Covid-19 pandemic, we have seen the way in which technology has become increasingly important, given mandates to social distance or self-isolate, and the need to engage and train a geographically disparate healthcare workforce. However, Winters et al. (2018) have argued that most deployments of digital training programmes adhere to over-simplified models of learning that fail to account for the complexities that emerge when new technologies are introduced into pedagogical practice. In response, chapter authors have advocated embedding pedagogical theory into digital initiatives during the design and implementation phases of training and supervision programmes, outlining the need for a paradigm shift away from the 'techno-deterministic design focus', towards one informed by context. Kelley and Fancourt (Chapter 11) have also suggested the need for a shift in training philosophy, whereby ethical principles should be incorporated into pedagogy from the outset.

Furthermore, Panjabi et al. (Chapter 2) draw attention to the complexity of any training or supervision programme that is supported by digital tools. There is a need for all aspects of a system—algorithm development, multimedia development, data collection tools etc.—to be coordinated or there will be a 'fragmented tool set and an unstable foundation for blended learning'. At present, there are silos existing between disciplines that directly inform CHW training, but our authors have underlined the value of interdisciplinary conversations, particularly when it comes to underpinning an intervention with pedagogical principles.

These discussions have placed learning pedagogy, understanding local context, and the empowerment of CHWs, at the very foreground of effective, ethical, and interdisciplinary training programmes for CHWs, and argue that participatory approaches are the most appropriate means to put these principles into practice.

Participatory Approaches

As previously noted, there has been a move beyond information dissemination and calls for a greater emphasis on participatory approaches so that programmes can be more sensitive and responsive to needs of CHWs and their communities (see O'Donovan, Chapter 4). Whilst there are a wide range of participatory methods that might be employed, each shares the aim to empower CHW trainees through critical (self)-reflection, seeks to equalize the relationship between trainers and trainees, to place value on participant experience, and to lay the essential foundations for continuous learning. A good example of this is given by Wasunna and Holeman (Chapter 5), who detail how a participatory approach led to the use of data to improve the process of face-to-face supervision, rather than developing technologies to replace the supervisor.

Participatory approaches go some way towards the commitment to social justice and relational ethics set out by Kelley and Fancourt (Chapter 11), in which these authors argue that the building of relationships and support can help to foster, successful, sustainable community health programmes. Musoke (Chapter 8) emphasizes that in choosing the most appropriate training methods to use in CHW programmes, it is important to consider several factors, such as the number, level of education, and experience of trainees; the resources available, including time, materials, and technology; as well as the topic and context of the training.

Evaluation and Evidence Mapping

If we are to learn from CHW training and supervision programmes, we must be able to provide evidence that their training is effective in preparing CHWs for their roles (or in maintaining or enhancing their knowledge and skills over time). The contributors to this volume have highlighted the acute challenges of monitoring and evaluation, particularly in low resource, and often geographically isolated settings. The choice of evaluation method is key, and there are important questions raised as to how to interpret outcome measures. Brown (Chapter 10) emphasizes that there is no 'one size fits all' approach to evaluation, and the appropriate choice will depend on the existing evidence regarding the training planned, the intended audience for the evaluation and the resources available for the evaluation.

Throughout this book, authors have argued for a clear, evidence-based understanding of what is required of CHWs that can inform training and supervision programmes. As emphasized by Nduku et al. (Chapter 9), initiatives need to be carefully reviewed, based on the existing evidence base, for their relevance, effectiveness, and equity implications in the contexts in which CHWs are operating. However, this remains an area in which the evidence relating to education approaches and supervision strategies is still underdeveloped (ibid). This lack of evidence-based educational practice guidelines presents a major barrier to the effective and equitable training of CHWs. Nduku et al. (Chapter 9) also emphasize that many training programmes for CHWs are not based on evidence that has been at least co-produced with CHWs themselves. A systematic practice of using a diverse range of evidence, especially evidence from CHWs, is an important step in efforts to design more effective and equitable programmes.

Drawing on all the chapters, what becomes evident is an increasing tendency to move away from mere top-down training programmes for CHWs towards participatory training and supervision approaches. However, as we have tried to argue through this volume, for *a truly just approach*, the focus now needs to shift towards removing any remaining obstacles and barriers that keep CHWs from being equitable stakeholders and partners in this endeavour. Only then will the move from historically influenced knowledge dissemination efforts, to more equitable training approaches, to a just and liberated, self-governed knowledge production by CHWs be complete, and a *pedagogy by and for CHWs established.*

Ways Forward

At a time of health crisis, such as the Covid-19 pandemic, CHWs find themselves at the front-line of detection, prevention, and response. In 2020, CHWs in Liberia conducted infection prevention and control measures, explained and promoted social distancing, organized hand hygiene stations, and educated their neighbours about interrupting disease transmission. There is a role for CHWs in supporting patients who are self-isolating and monitoring them in the community, while ensuring delivery of food, social, and medical support—a form of accompaniment (Palazuelos et al., 2018). CHWs supported the monitoring of patients for clinical deterioration and supported the rapid referral of individuals who required hospitalization, reinforcing links between the health system and communities (as undertaken by Muso in Mali). And, CHWs supported contact tracing, symptom reporting, and monitoring the contacts of patients with Covid-19 to ensure access to testing and treatment for those who developed signs and symptoms (ibid.). Finally, CHWs can sustain primary healthcare services that would otherwise be interrupted, providing care protocols are updated (e.g. by introducing physical distancing and using appropriate personal protective equipment during patient encounters) so that CHWs remain safe, well supervised, and at reduced risk of transmitting SARS-CoV-2 (Wiah et al., 2020).

Yet, as this volume has argued, all of these vital functions must be supported by effective and adaptable training and supervisory tools, programmes and protocols that are not only informed by evidence and pedagogical theory but are empowering and ethical in their foundations. Furthermore, the increasingly digital operation of CHW health training, and health systems in general, means the training content cannot be seen in isolation from related data collection, diagnostic applications, telehealth for referrals, and opportunities for peer-based learning that necessarily fall into a CHW's remit. The contributing authors in this volume have suggested some ways forward to support these challenging but laudable ambitions.

The first of these is the use of human-centred design or participatory design approaches to create training programmes. Wasunna and Holemann (Chapter 5) discuss the way in which a human centred design approach to training and supervision of CHWs led to a deeper understanding of the contextual factors that are likely to influence design, uptake, and sustainability of digital health interventions. By co-creating with the end user, the authors argued they were able to identify training models that are suitable and sustainable to the context in which these digital health interventions are deployed. Attending more broadly to human experience in this way involves looking beyond the design of discrete technologies to reimagine services, the organization of health systems, and broader social arrangements that pattern who receives equitable care and who does not. This relates to calls for a stronger ethical agenda in the pedagogical underpinnings of CHW training and supervision. Kelley and Fancourt (Chapter 11) call for relational pedagogy for training and supervision outlined to address some key values: mutual respect and recognition; shared decision-making and solidarity; relational agency and empowerment; fairness and inclusion; and shared advocacy.

In order to better understand the effectiveness, transferability, and external validity of individual CHWs training programmes, Nduku et al. (Chapter 9) argue for systematically collated and appraised evidence mapping. Evidence maps seek to provide a policy- and practice-relevant evidence base, placing a much stronger emphasis on user engagement compared to traditional systematic reviews. Their production requires interdisciplinary cooperation between government and the research sector.

Finally, in recognition of the need to move beyond small-scale, pilot-style CHW projects to widespread sustainable health workforce systems, Panjabi et al. (Chapter 2) suggest a strong rationale for a globally representative and locally adaptable CHW curriculum which can be contextualized for local need as required. This is coupled with the efficiencies of digital technology and increasingly clear commonalities of the necessary curriculum. There is thus a great need for international and interdisciplinary coordination. In their detailed and informative case study, Last Mile Health set out the crucial steps to establish this sort of cooperative relationship, and highlight some of the biggest obstacles they have encountered.

This volume has sought to provide a resource to inform practitioners, policymakers, and academics alike. With a balance of theoretical discussion and practical detail, enhanced with the rich case studies presented in the book, we hope to have highlighted the importance of collaboration between disciplines and organizations. In recognition of a rapidly changing field, we have provided online resources that may allow the reader to keep up to date more easily (www.mhealthpartners.org/book). Together, we have set out a roadmap for efforts to shape new CHW-driven pedagogies, embodying a shift from equality, to equity, to ultimately justice and liberation.

References

Bhutta, Z., Lassi, Z.S., Pariyo, G., & Huicho, L. (2010). Global experience of community health workers for delivery of health related millennium developmental goals: A systematic review, country case studies, and recommendations for integration into national health systems. Geneva, World Health Organization. Available from: http://www.who.int/workforcealliance/knowledge/publications/alliance/Global_CHW_web.pdf

Heymann, D.L., Chen, L., Takemi, K., Fidler, D.P., Tappero, J.W., Thomas, M.J., et al. (2015). Global health security: The wider lessons from the west African Ebola virus disease epidemic. *Lancet*, 385(9980), 1884–1901. DOI: 10.1016/S0140-6736(15)60858-3.

Palazuelos, D., Farmer, P., & Mukherjee, J. (2018). Community health and equity of outcomes: The Partners in Health experience. *Lancet*, 6(5), e491–e493.

Perry, H.B., Zulliger, R., & Rogers, M.M. (2014). Community health workers in low-, middle-, and high-income countries: An overview of their history, recent evolution, and current effectiveness. *Annual Review of Public Health*, 35(1), 399–421.

Perry, H.B., Dhillon, R.S., Liu, A., Chitnis, K., Panjabi, R., Palazuelos, D., et al. (2016). Community health worker programmes after the 2013–2016 Ebola outbreak. *Bulletin of the World Health Organization*, 94(7), 551–553.

Schaaf, M., Fox, J., Topp, S.M., Warthin, C., Freedman, L., Sullivan Robinson, R., et al. (2018). Community health workers and accountability: Reflections from an international 'think-in'. *International Journal for Equity in Health*, 17(66). https://doi.org/10.1186/s12939-018-0781-5

Vandi, M.A., van Griensven, J., Chan, A.K., Kargbo, B., Kandeh, J.N., Alpha, K.S., et al. (2017). Ebola and community health worker services in Kenema District, Sierra Leone: Please mind the gap! *Public Health Action*, 7(1), S55–S61. doi:10.5588/pha.16.0082.

Wiah, O.S., Subah, M., Varpilah, B., Waters, A., Ly, J., Ballard, M., et al. (2020). Prevent, detect, respond: How community health workers can help in the fight against covid-19. *BMJ Opinion*. Available from: https://blogs.bmj.com/bmj/2020/03/27/prevent-detect-respond-how-community-health-workers-can-help-fight-covid-19/

Winters, N., Langer, L., Nduku, P., Robson, J., O'Donovan, J., Maulik, P., Paton, C., Geniets, A., Peiris, D., & Nagraj, S. (2019). Using mobile technologies to support the training of community health workers in low-income and middle-income countries: mapping the evidence. *BMJ Global Health*, 4(4), e001421.

Afterword
Pedagogy of the Technical and the Political

Ṣẹ̀yẹ Abímbọ́lá

Whenever I am confronted with the need to make sense of a health system issue, I sort the actors involved according to the rules that govern their actions, decisions, and relations—and according to the rules that they make, change, monitor, and enforce. In this analytic framing, everyone is a health system actor (Abimbola et al., 2017; 2020a). Everyone in a community. But also, everyone involved outside the community, as long as their actions, decisions, and relations affect health within the community of interest. Wherever they are located, these actors function within what one may describe as 'three worlds of action' (Kiser & Ostrom, 1982), 'three levels of governance' (Abimbola et al., 2014), or 'three levels of rules' (McGinnis, 2011)—namely: operational, collective, and constitutional—sorted into a triangle (Abimbola, 2020b). See Figure A1.

The first level of governance, that is, the *operational level*, contains rules that emerge from individual choices and the market forces of demand and supply. They determine

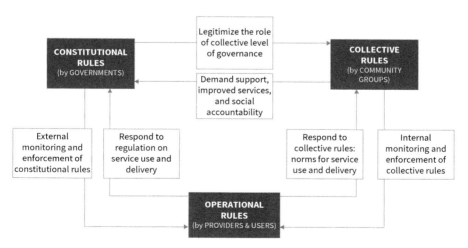

Figure A1 The 'triangle of rules' (Abimbola, 2020b) showing bi-directional relations between each of the nodes of the triangle with the other two nodes, using the example of rules that govern service delivery within a community.

Ṣẹ̀yẹ Abímbọ́lá, *Afterword* In: *Training for Community Health*. Edited by: Anne Geniets, James O'Donovan, Laura Hakimi, and Niall Winters, Oxford University Press. © Oxford University Press 2021. DOI: 10.1093/oso/9780198866244.003.0013

how individual actors implement practical day-to-day decisions; how, for example, market rules (in the form of prices), informal rules (e.g. social norms), and formal rules (e.g. government regulations) determine how people in a community seek, use (i.e. demand), and provide (i.e. supply) health services (Kiser & Ostrom, 1982; McGinnis, 2011; Abimbola et al., 2014; Abimbola, 2020a). In my mental map, I had always positioned community health workers (CHWs) primarily, if not exclusively, as operational actors, on both supply and demand sides (Abimbola et al., 2014). That was until I read a paper four years ago, in which members of 'community health committees' were placed on a list of people who may be described as CHWs (Baatiema et al., 2016). Once I considered such re-framing, it seemed immediately obvious. Notably, 'community health committees' are the most common form by which community engagement in primary health care governance has been promoted in global health (McCoy et al., 2011; Molyneux et al., 2012).

Existing in varying forms across sub-Saharan Africa, and from Central and South America to Central, South, and South East Asia, these committees are named differently in various settings—as village, ward, or community health committees, as development committees, or health facility management or governing committees (McCoy et al., 2011). Their significant overlap with the people who are typically referred to as CHWs is clear when you consider their membership, which also varies from place to place. They include influential community members, the health worker in charge of the health facility to which the committee is linked, representatives of traditional, voluntary, religious, women, and youth groups; of informal health care providers (e.g. traditional healers, traditional birth attendants, and patent medicine vendors); and of relevant non-health occupational groups (e.g. school headteachers and workers in the electricity and water sectors) (McCoy et al., 2011; Abimbola et al., 2016a; 2016b; Abimbola, 2020a). For some reason, I had framed 'community health committees' as a separate kind of entity, distinct from CHWs. They are at the collective level of governance (Abimbola et al., 2014).

The second level of governance, that is, the *collective level*, contains the rules that influence day-to-day demand and supply side operational activities, typically made by 'close-to-ground' governing entities, which may be informal or formally constituted. Examples of 'close-to-ground' governing entities on the demand side may include groups of community representatives, such as traditional cultural groups, religious groups, and women's groups. And on the supply side, 'close-to-ground' governing entities may include locally-based professional groups, for example of midwives or traditional birth attendants (Kiser & Ostrom, 1982; McGinnis, 2011; Abimbola et al., 2014; Abimbola, 2020a). Notably, these examples on either the demand or supply sides can be flipped vice versa. Members of 'community health committees' function at this level—after all their main role was to co-manage primary health care within their community; making, changing, monitoring, and enforcing the rules that govern operational actors (Abimbola et al., 2017; Abimbola, 2020a). What is not clear is that CHWs can be operational and collective actors, depending on their role.

Indeed, governing roles are enacted through a range of modes in which the community health committees function (Abimbola et al., 2016a; 2016b; Abimbola, 2020a)—for example as 'village square' (by being a forum through which community members meet to discuss and address health challenges); as 'community connectors' (by reaching out in their community, to connect community members to their service providers, and demanding social accountability from such providers); as 'government botherers' (by lobbying and demanding social accountability from governments); as 'back-up government' (by augmenting government support, and by seeking support community members, non-government organizations (NGOs), and other non-government sources); and as 'general overseers' (by taking control of the supply of health services in their community, especially when governments fail). In other words, like other CHWs, 'community health committees' can function as service extenders, cultural brokers, and social or political change agents (Schaaf et al., 2020). Performing such a mix of roles effectively requires training, which is often lacking, especially for their roles as 'social or political change agents'. Yet, further constraining their ability to function as 'social or political change agents' is lack of legitimation for such roles by governments (Molyneux et al., 2012; George et al., 2015; Abimbola et al., 2016a; Abimbola, 2020a).

The third level of governance, that is, the *constitutional level*, contains rules that determine how collective rules are made, changed, monitored, and enforced. These are the rules that can legitimize the governance role of entities such as 'community health committees'. Constitutional rules can determine who has the power to make collective and operational rules and on what terms they do so. Constitutional rules can also determine how rules at the collective and operational levels are made, changed, monitored, and enforced. In addition, constitutional rules may directly influence operational rules. And constitutional rules may also influence operational rules, indirectly through how they influence collective rules (Kiser & Ostrom, 1982; McGinnis, 2011; Abimbola et al., 2014; Abimbola, 2020a). Constitutional rules are made, typically at a distance, by governments and government-like entities such as large and influential NGOs or religious organizations with national (or large-scale) jurisdiction and reach (Kiser & Ostrom, 1982; McGinnis, 2011; Abimbola et al., 2014; Abimbola, 2020a).

The broad range of roles performed by CHWs implies that their pedagogical needs is twofold—the pedagogy of the technical, to support their roles as service extenders and cultural brokers; and the pedagogy of the political, to support their roles as social or political change agents. Alongside technical knowledge and skills, they must also gain political knowledge and skills—especially for their relations with other actors in their community (e.g. how to build community coalitions to solve problems, how to demand social accountability from health professionals, and how to generate the local legitimacy necessary for such activities, say, by leveraging the authority of entities with power in the community, such as women's religious and traditional leaders); and with actors outside their community (e.g. how to know and demand their rights and entitlements, including the minimum standard of service provision to expect from the government, and how to ensure that their voices are heard beyond their community, especially at the constitutional level) (George et al., 2015; Abimbola et al., 2016a; 2016b; Abimbola, 2020a; Schaaf et al., 2020).

Notably, strategies to deliver such political training can be extrapolated from what is already covered in this book. Relevant for both kinds of pedagogy are, for example, the use of digital technologies, participatory methods, and human-centred design to integrate digital and face-to-face education and support; and a focus on relational expertise, and the 'hidden curriculum' of the peculiarities of how each community functions. However, the pedagogy of the political requires additional, and more focused, strategies. So far under-developed, those strategies will have to be underpinned by a rights-based approach, and a recognition that addressing social and political challenges is no less important than solving pressing technical problems.

References

Abimbola, S., Negin, J., Jan, S., & Martiniuk, A. (2014). Towards people-centred health systems: A multi-level framework for analysing primary health care governance in low- and middle-income countries. *Health Policy & Planning*, 29(Suppl. 2), ii29–39.

Abimbola, S., Molemodile, S.K., Okonkwo, O.A., Negin, J., Jan, S., Martiniuk, A.L. (2016a). 'The government cannot do it all alone': Realist analysis of the minutes of community health committee meetings in Nigeria. *Health Policy & Planning*, 31(3), 332–345.

Abimbola, S., Ogunsina, K., Charles-Okoli, A.N., Negin, J., Martiniuk, A.L., & Jan, S. (2016b). Information, regulation and coordination: Realist analysis of the efforts of community health committees to limit informal health care providers in Nigeria. *Health Economics Review*, 6, 51.

Abimbola, S., Negin, J., Martiniuk, A.L., & Jan, S. (2017). Institutional analysis of health system governance. *Health Policy & Planning*, 32(9), 1337–1344.

Abimbola, S. (2020a). Beyond positive a priori bias: Reframing community engagement in LMICs. *Health Promotion International*, 35(3), 598–609.

Abimbola, S. (2020b). Health system governance: A triangle of rules. *BMJ Global Health*, 5(8), e003598.

Baatiema, L., Sumah, A.M., Tang, P.N., & Ganle, J.K. (2016). Community health workers in Ghana: The need for greater policy attention. *BMJ Global Health*, 1(4), e000141.

George, A., Scott, K., Garimella, S., Mondal, S., Ved, R., & Sheikh, K. (2015). Anchoring contextual analysis in health policy and systems research: A narrative review of contextual factors influencing health committees in low and middle income countries. *Social Science & Medicine*, 133, 159–167.

Kiser, L.L. & Ostrom, E. (1982). The three worlds of action: A metatheoretical synthesis of institutional approaches. In: E. Ostrom (Ed.). *Strategies of Political Inquiry*. Beverly Hills, CA, Sage, pp. 179–222.

McCoy, D. C., Hall, J.A., & Ridge, M. (2011). A systematic review of the literature for evidence on health facility committees in low- and middle-income countries. *Health Policy & Planning*, 27(6), 449–466.

McGinnis, M.D. (2011). An introduction to IAD and the language of the Ostrom workshop: A simple guide to a complex framework. *Policy Studies Journal*, 39(1), 169–183.

Molyneux, S., Atela, M., Angwenyi, V., & Goodman, C. (2012). Community accountability at peripheral health facilities: A review of the empirical literature and development of a conceptual framework. *Health Policy & Planning*, 27(7), 541–554.

Schaaf, M., Warthin, C., Freedman, L., & Topp, S.M. (2020). The community health worker as service extender, cultural broker and social change agent: A critical interpretive synthesis of roles, intent and accountability. *BMJ Global Health*, 5(6), e002296.

The Community Health Academy Initiative at LMH

A Collaborative Approach to Develop a Blended Learning Curriculum for Health Workers

https://lastmilehealth.org/what-we-do/
community-health-academy/

Organisational Profile

Founded on the belief that no one should die because of distance from a health worker, Last Mile Health (LMH) partners with governments to design and scale national networks of front-line and community health workers (CHWs) that deliver life-saving essential healthcare services to their neighbours' doorsteps. Working alongside the Liberian Ministry of Health (LMH) is advancing universal health coverage in Liberia by supporting scale-up of Liberia's National Community Health Assistant Program, which will deploy a network of over 4000 community and front-line health workers to serve all 1.2 million rural people in Liberia by the end of 2021. Building on lessons learned in Liberia, LMH now partners with governments in Ethiopia, Malawi, Sierra Leone and Uganda to strengthen the quality of their community health systems through technical advising, training, policy, and research. Over the next four years, LMH will accelerate the global movement for community-based primary healthcare by supporting at least 16,000 community and front-line health workers to serve over nine million rural people and will share its methods globally. To date, LMH has secured the majority of its funding from private philanthropists. The organization has also partnered with bi- and multilateral donors such as USAID's Development Innovation Program (DIV) and Gavi, the Vaccine Alliance.

The Academy Initiative

LMH is working closely with the Federal Ministry of Health in Ethiopia (FMOH) to use digital technologies to modernize the approach to health worker training at the community level.

Using the Ethiopia Health Extension Worker (HEW) curriculum as the starting point, LMH, under the leadership of the FMHO, and working with other partners, proposes to leverage the use of mobile technology to provide health workers access to high-quality, multi-media educational content that complements content provided through face-to-face training.

What makes this work distinctive is that it is not a 'one-off' project that will require long-term engagement of external 'experts' providing technical assistance to the FMOH. The approach is designed to ensure that both the content development and delivery process is owned and managed by the Ministry. This approach requires partnering with organizations willing to give up ownership of the content and the process and buy in to a shared vision that genuinely puts health system development in the hands of the country.

Establishing a Partnership

Partnerships, collaboration, and government ownership of community health systems strengthening are values that underpin LMH's work. LMH took the following steps to establish its partnership with the FMOH in Ethiopia. These steps chart the route to engagement and partnership with other countries who can draw from and adapt a similar approach to support their own health workforce strengthening strategies:

1. *Start with government*: LMH's mandate to address the challenge of providing quality health worker training on a global basis stemmed from a Technology, Entertainment, Design (TED) talk delivered by Dr Raj Panjabi, LMH's CEO, in 2017. Dr Panjabi highlighted the advancements in technology that allow health workers to access health information and training in an accessible multi-media format. This led to a meeting with the Minister of Health in Ethiopia, which became the first step in an 18-month sequence of conversations and meetings culminating in an agreement with FMOH to develop a blended learning curriculum, using the Ethiopia HEW curriculum as the starting point.

2. *Create a vision*: the challenges of delivering effective and timely health worker training at the community level, and the potential for digital technologies to address those challenges, is well documented in the previous chapter. It would be tempting to simply create a global digital library of health education videos that could be downloaded onto a health worker's phone and then periodically update these videos or adapt them to new circumstances. A simple solution to a complex problem. However, such a solution—which has been tried before—does not lead to the sustainable change that governments are seeking. Such a solution ignores the vitally important and multiple interconnections between the content, the health worker, the individual health system within a country, existing standards, guidelines and protocols, country ownership of the product and process, feedback mechanisms to gauge the effectiveness of the content, sustainability of the inevitable change and adaption process for the content and the technology that delivers it, interoperability of the delivery system with other health worker support technologies, and much more.

3. *Create shared ownership of the vision*: the next step will be to work with partners who viewed the challenge—and proposed solution—in the same way. Embracing a systems thinking approach required many conversations—both virtual and in person—between implementing partners, funders, and others. It was clear that if the Academy's proposal to develop a blended learning curriculum was to gain traction across sub-Saharan Africa (and more widely), it would have to first partner with a country that would be a reliable point of reference for other countries across the continent.

4. *Establish the foundational ministry of health partnership*: the Ethiopia HEW programme had already been recognized, by WHO, health ministries in several African countries, multi- and bi-lateral donors, UNICEF, and others, as a model to be emulated more widely to improve health outcomes at the community level. Since the initial discussion had already taken place between Dr Panjabi and the Minister of Health, it made sense for LMH to further engage with the FMOH to assess its interest in being a foundational government partner in the development of the blended learning curriculum. Over the next 18 months, a series of meetings and workshops took place with representatives from the FMOH, as well as with implementing partners, donors, and others working on community health systems strengthening in Ethiopia. The culmination of these meetings was an invitation by the FMOH to LMH to create a multi-stakeholder partnership to develop a blended learning curriculum, using the Ethiopia HEW curriculum as a starting point.

5. *Create the multi-stakeholder partnership*: designing and developing a blended learning curriculum, once support from FMOH staff and implementing partners has been secured, requires expertise in a number of areas including: digital technology, multimedia

production, clinical and behavioral medicine, curriculum development, and a deep understanding of the pedagogical approaches that work for training health workers at the community level. LMH identified organizations that already had knowledge and experience in each of these areas and, more importantly, believed in the vision. They were willing to set aside organizational priorities and agree to collaborate towards the common goal of creating both a product and a sustainable process that would be recognized as a global public good.

6. *Establish areas of expertise to create the content and delivery process*: the areas of expertise required were broken down into three components:
   - Multi-media creation: to compensate for the quality gap in performance and outcomes, create multimedia for in-service training designed for local production accessing global expertise where appropriate.
   - Establish a digital network model: by converting existing and new materials into a digital format Ministries can: shorten the amount of time required to train CHWs; reduce the number of trainers required to teach CHWs; and create content that is easier and cheaper to standardize and disseminate. Taken together, these advantages imply drastic reductions in the cost of training the one million new CHWs that Sub-Saharan Africa needs while ensuring that content is up to date and traceable to standards.
   - Partner with a technology provider: Digital Campus has created a proven, open source technology for content delivery which is designed for country ownership: Oppia Mobile. Oppia Mobile can process and deliver content offline to users, record, and forward analytics concerning content usage and knowledge, and interoperate with approved existing and proposed systems. As such, it provides a pathway for government ownership.

7. *Agree the partnerships and develop the workplan*: the culmination of negotiations with implementing partners, led to an agreement between the FMOH and LMH to move ahead with developing the blended learning curriculum starting with RMNCH.

8. *Scale up across sub-Saharan Africa*: at the same time that discussions were taking place with the FMOH and partners in Ethiopia, LMH was engaging with ministries of health in several other countries in sub-Saharan Africa. These countries (including Liberia, Uganda, and Sierra Leone) have signalled their interest in adapting a blended learning curriculum. These conversations, combined with ongoing advocacy efforts, constitute the first steps of the process to create what LMH and its partners hope will evolve into an initiative that moves beyond the typical project orientation towards sustainable, government-led community health systems and health workforce strengthening.

Practical Tips for Success

1. *If the evidence and the principal partner (in this case the FMOH) support a solution, don't compromise on its implementation.* Instead, work closely with the partner and wider community to socialize the solution and create buy-in. This takes time, perseverance, and patience, all of which can appear to slow down progress. Seeing relationships and consensus-building as a critical part of the process is important and needs to be integrated into planning from the start.

2. *Achieving real collaboration is more important than advancing innovations.* Too often the rapid implementation of singular, innovative ideas and/or technologies comes at the cost of key partnerships which ultimately prevent scaling potential solutions. Working with countries with evidence of political will and capacity to expand and sustain a solution is more likely to lead to improved community health outcomes at scale.

Key Challenges

1. *Securing partnerships in advance of implementation.* If you are in start-up mode and insist upon relying on fully vetted, in-house hires to implement the bulk of activities associated with such an initiative you are likely to be disappointed with both the pace of implementation and its outcome. Although finding the right partner can be as challenging as finding the right employee, partnering with an organization that has a proven track record and is already trusted by the governments you are working with, speeds up the time in getting all the players to mesh in an effective, cohesive manner.
2. *Donor coordination and building a shared vision.* Working with multiple donors to develop and advance a global public good (something many donors have no experience with) can create governance challenges. Furthermore, a programme involving technology does not mean that indicators such as 'number of modules deployed' or 'number of health workers equipped with mobile devices' will adequately reflect the status of the programme, despite these being the kinds of metrics donors often expect to see. It is therefore important to emphasize the systems-based approach and build a shared vision with the donors for the broader projected impact of your programme.
3. *Leverage the commonality of training content and the flexibility of a digital format to share common practices and products where possible.* Despite the commonality in CHW training content, and the need to ensure traceability of training materials to original guidelines and protocols, nearly every health ministry around the world periodically recreates training materials from scratch. Despite the logic and potential savings that could result from sharing common practices and products, the institutions that have established an existing approach towards health worker training are unlikely to change any time soon. Ministries may recognize the value of transitioning to an approach that recognizes the value of sharing common resources but are locked into a digital and health worker ecosystem that has little incentive to change. LMH will continue to advocate for change while working to combine digital technology with traditional face-to-face methods for a more effective and economical blended learning approach to health worker training.

LEAP

The mHealth Platform

https://amrefuk.org/what-we-do/projects/
leap-the-mhealth-platform/

Organizational Profile

Country of operation: amref Health Africa operates in Kenya with country offices in ten African
countries including: Tanzania, Uganda, Ethiopia, South Sudan, and Malawi. Its project reach
is serving millions of people in 35 African countries.

Number of CHWs: 3000 community health volunteers (CHVs) had been trained using the
LEAP mobile platform by 2017 in 13 counties in Kenya. These are: Nairobi, Kisumu, Siaya,
Kakamega, Bungoma, Vihiga, Kisii, Migori, Nyamira, Kitui, Kajiado, Isiolo, and Samburu.

Partnership model: amref Health Africa has worked in a public–private partnership with
Accenture, the Kenyan Ministry of Health, SAFARICOM (which provided the telecommunications infrastructure to deliver LEAP in remote areas) and Mezzanine (which developed
the technology).

CHW Cadre

Name given to CHWs: CHVs.

Recruitment: CHVs are selected by the community and they work voluntarily to provide important links to the health system. Health non-governmental organizations (NGOs) support their work through provision of allowance during project activities and equipment.
Depending on the region, CHVs are respected members of the community with some basic
education.

Responsibility: each CHV covers approximately 100 households.

Traditional CHV Training

Expansion of the formal health system to communities and households impacts multiple levels
of healthcare in Kenya as the household is perceived to be the first care unit and the CHVs as
the first level care providers. Recognizing the need to strengthen community health systems by
introducing innovative programmes that capacity build the CHVs is key in enhancing effective
service delivery at community level. Kenya adopted CHVs as its own resource persons to provide services in the community, who are selected by the community and work voluntarily.

The Ministry under the Division of Community Health Services developed a handbook
for training CHVs (MOH, 2013). The manual has six core modules that cover the following
areas: (1) health and development; (2) community governance and leadership; (3) communication, advocacy, and social mobilization; (4) best practices for health promotion and diseases prevention; (5) basic healthcare and life-saving skills; and (6) management and use of

community health information and disease surveillance. The manual has been used by different organizations to train CHVs using face-to-face approaches through seminars and workshops that typically last a few days.

LEAP formally known as the Health Enablement and Learning Platform (HELP) was a three-phase project funded by Accenture Global Giving and M-PESA Foundation. The project targeted the training of both the new and existing CHVs and community health extension workers (CHEWs).

The project addressed the need of the Ministry of Health (MOH) to train, upskill, and develop the capacity of CHVs and their supervisors (CHEWs), who are a critical component in delivering community health services across Kenya. The project was implemented in three phases, of which phase 1 was testing and took 12 months; phase II covered a 24-month period that ran from September 2014 to August 2016. These papers addressed the outcome by the end of phase II, where the aim was to scale-up mobile training from 300 achieved in phase I to 3000 across three different socio-economic regions (nomadic, rural, and urban).

Typically, CHVs are trained by traditional face-to-face classroom training. Amref Health has noted that this has three particular challenges:

- Poor knowledge retention after health workers have been trained, with no easy way to revisit training modules.
- High attrition due to low ongoing health worker engagement.
- Inability to rapidly connect and mobilize health workers in an outbreak.

The mHealth Platform

In order to attain the targeted scale-up, the LEAP project endeavoured to develop, enhance, and deploy CHV mLearning content, integrate with third party applications, and measure the health and skills outcomes associated with mLearning. LEAP is an integrated mobile health platform that uses regular updates and peer-to-peer communication to increase the knowledge and strengthen the skills of health workers.

mLearning complements initial face-to-face training, enabling the CHVs to learn at their own pace, at their own time using their own mobile devices while in their communities. LEAP delivers approved MOH curricula and more, through a combination of text and audio messages, making it accessible through basic mobile phones.

The platform allowed for content to be delivered in English and Kiswahili (local language) languages which supported learning for CHV with different levels of formal education. This supported decisions at the community level through diagnostic trees.

Format of Training

CHVs receive initial face-to-face training and later gain access to the mLearning platform. CHVs receive training content through their mobile phones in the 29 topics on the platform.

The topics have been drawn from the six core modules in the CHV developed by MOH for as follows:

- Health and development.
- Community governance and leadership.
- Communication, advocacy, and social mobilization.
- Best practices for health promotion and disease prevention.
- Basic healthcare and life saving skills.
- Management of community health information and disease surveillance.

Monthly feedback sessions were held with each of the community units (CUs) enrolled on the system to share feedback and experiences in mLearning as well as deal with any issues that may be affecting their performance in mLearning. Some of the issues affecting completion of the topics included poor network coverage in the areas and instability in the platform, resulting in SMS delays and IVR drops. During the feedback sessions, the learners were encouraged to begin their topics as soon as they received them to ensure they maintained the interest in the topic. Learners were also encouraged to chat about the topics of the week, using the LEAP group chat feature, to motivate the slow learners to catch up with fast learners. The project also used a 'learning buddy' system where slow learners are grouped with the faster learners to ensure that there is closer support and motivation to learn and complete the topics.

Learners' progress is monitored through evaluations, quizzes, and practical exercises, as well as real-time performance reports and supervision tools. Supervisors of CHVs can also access CHV progress.

Training Outcomes

Training evaluations have noted:

- Improved CHV engagement and reduced attrition.
- Better CHV knowledge retention.
- Strengthened community health unit cohesiveness.
- Faster responses and mobilizations to outbreaks.
- LEAP mHealth platform is now available to other partners for use in strengthening their CHV training programmes.

Practical Tips for Success

- Supervision and partners support to help engagement and to avoid attrition.
- Motivation of CHVs through allowances.
- Constant engagement of CHVs is important and promotes continued education.

Reference

Kenyan Ministry of Health (2013). *Community Health Volunteers Handbook*. Nairobi, Kenya: MOH.

Muso

www.musohealth.org

Organizational Profile

Country of operation: Mali

Number of CHWs: 431 community health workers (CHWs) across rural and peri-urban Mali.

Funders: Muso receives funding from over 40 different partners, including Child Relief International, the Bill & Melinda Gates Foundation, Grand Challenges Canada, and many others.

Partnership model: Muso partners directly with Mali's Ministry of Health, from national to local. In both Yirimadio and Bankass, Muso partners with the local community health associations to recruit, train, and supervise CHWs. CHWs sign their contracts directly with their community health associations, and their payment and benefits are all managed by the associations; Muso reimburses the community health associations for CHW salaries and benefits.

CHW Cadre

Remuneration: Muso's *CHWs are salaried*, receiving 40,000 FCFA per month, or approximately $75 USD. They also *receive benefits* in the form of social security and health insurance.

Recruitment: the recruitment process is managed from start to finish by a small recruitment committee, convened by the community health association.

CHW criteria: age 18–45; able to read and write in the primary working language (Bamanankan in Yirimadio, French in Bankass); able to communicate verbally in the majority language (Bamanankan in Yirimadio, Dogon, Peuhl, or Bamanankan in Bankass); motivated to do the work; resident of the community to be served. All else being equal, preference is given to female candidates.

Education requirements: Muso does not have an education or diploma requirement. In Mali, educational achievement often functions as a proxy for male sex and socioeconomic privilege, and the organization has not found diploma status to be a good predictor of CHW performance. Instead, such requirements have the effect of unnecessarily excluding qualified female candidates.

Accreditation: Muso does not have a formal accreditation process for CHWs, rather it relies on the initial training, annual refresher trainings, and the 360 degree supervision model for quality control of CHW performance.

Training Approach

Muso's learning and innovations team has developed its own CHW recruitment and training procedures and training manuals, which are aligned with and build off the national standards. Muso's learning and innovations team runs a 'train the trainers' training with that team of technical staff to prepare them to give the trainings using Muso's manuals and procedures. The training takes a total of 36 days, broken into two 18-day sessions. Training groups average 20 candidate CHWs per group.

The training covers the following topics:

- Healthcare as a human right; social justice.
- The fundamental roles, responsibilities, and tasks of a CHW.
- The importance of proactive CHW workflow.
- Safety while working as a CHW.
- 360 degree supervision.
- The Muso-Medic CHW App: how to use the smartphone, how to use the App to support daily workflows, how to submit data via the App.

The trainings are designed to be extremely interactive, with minimal 'lecturing'. When learning to use the CHW App, candidates have phones in hand and use the App exactly as it's used in the field.

CHWs are evaluated as follows:

- A written test that evaluates comprehension of the CHW protocols.
- An evaluation of each candidate by the trainers. The trainers rate each candidate on five different criteria: communication abilities, nature of their participation during the training, attitude towards learning during the training, problem-solving capacity, active listening.

360 Degree Supervision

Muso's model of CHW supervision is called 360 degree supervision. CHW supervisors are recruited into full-time salaried positions and provided with an initial six-day training. Their training provides in-depth orientation on a structured model of supportive supervision, an overview of the protocol that CHWs follow, and instruction on the use of a CHW supervisor App. Thereafter they provide dedicated supervision to a cohort of 15 to 20 CHWs (average 18). Supervisors are additionally equipped with tablets, a tablet based CHW supervisor App, and a motorcycle.

The 360 degree supervision model consists of four key elements:

- *Group supervision meetings.* Each supervisor holds in-person group meetings with their cohort on a weekly (in a peri-urban setting) or bi-weekly (in a rural setting) basis.
- *Patient feedback audit.* The supervisor begins by visiting patient homes alone in order to collect patient feedback and verify reporting.
- *CHW shadowing.* Next, the supervisor finds the CHW to shadow her while she makes door-to-door rounds in her community.
- *One-on-one feedback.* The visit ends with a 1:1 sit down discussion. The supervisor begins by giving the CHW a chance to speak about their work: what does the CHW view as her own strengths and areas for improvement. The supervisor then provides summary feedback based on three data sources: the patient feedback audit, the direct shadowing, and the CHW dashboard, which provides summary analytics on the CHW's performance over time (see below). Together, the CHW and supervisor identify areas of strength to reinforce and areas requiring improvement.

Practical Tips For Success

- Co-create training content with the end users. Much of what Muso does today comes from feedback from several generations of CHW cohorts.

- Use CHW data to identify systemic practice issues and be prepared to use those lessons to adjust training manuals.
- Initial training is not enough. CHWs need ongoing, dedicated, supportive supervision to be successful. Muso has also found annual refresher trainings to be essential.
- Use CHW supervisors to surface common and recurring practice challenges that need to be re-visited in annual refresher trainings and reworked in the initial training materials.
- If something isn't working, conduct direct observations in the community and then workshops to find the solution with CHWs and their supervisors.

Muso and Medic: The CHW Dashboard

Medic worked with Muso to design a CHW dashboard that provides precision feedback on the care that each CHW provides. The dashboard displays an individual CHW's coverage, speed, and quality of care indicators from the previous month, using absolute numbers, percentages, and visual graphics, alongside those of the highest performing CHW. During the individual supervisory feedback session, this personalized and relative (to the highest performer) quantitative performance feedback helps orient the discussion of strengths and weaknesses and allows the CHW to see quantitatively and visually how his/her performance fared the previous month. The feedback provided to CHWs is both quantitative, informed by the dashboard, and qualitative, informed by the patient perspectives (supervision without CHW), and direct observation (supervision with CHW).

Following deployment of the supervisor dashboard, Muso, Medic, and the Malian Ministry of Health undertook a randomized controlled trial (RCT) with the aim of assessing the effects of the personalized performance dashboard used as a supervision tool, involving 148 CHWs conducting proactive case-finding home visits in Yirimadio, Mali (Whidden et al., 2018). Of these 148 CHWS, 73 were randomly allocated to receive individual monthly supervision with the CHW performance dashboard and an additional 75 received individual monthly supervision.

The results of this RCT highlights a range of key findings. These include:

- Pre-and post-intervention comparisons of the number of CHW homes visits, timeliness, and quality of CHW care showed improvements in the three outcomes over the study period.
- A 17% point increase was observed in children <5 years of age treated without protocol errors (quality) in the post-intervention (67%) when compared to the pre-intervention period (50%).
- The quantity (544 vs. 504), timeliness (87% vs. 83%), and quality (71 vs. 63%) of CHWS in the intervention arm was better when compared to the control group.
- When the analysis was restricted to the CHWs who received individual monthly supervision with the performance dashboard there was a significant increase in the average number of CHW home visits per month, by almost 40 visits (95% CI = 3.56–76.3), without compromising the quality or timeliness of care.

Reference

Whidden, C., Kayentao, K., Liu, J.X., Lee, S., Keita, Y., Diakité, D., et al. (2018). Improving community health worker performance by using a personalised feedback dashboard for supervision: A randomised controlled trial. *Journal of Global Health*, 8(2), 020418.

Partners in Health

https://www.pih.org/

Organizational Profile

Country of operation: Partners in Health (PIH) works across ten countries: Haiti (central plateau and St Marc), Mexico (southern Chiapas), Peru (Carabayllo), Navajo Nation, Rwanda (Southern Kayonza, Kirehe, Burera), Malawi (Neno), Lesotho (nearly national), Liberia (Maryland, Grand Gedeh), Sierra Leone (Kono), Kazakhstan.

Number of CHWs: >11,000 community health workers (CHWs) across ten countries.

Organizational history: PIH started in the late 1980s in Haiti, Peru in the 1990s, and then expanded to Rwanda, Malawi, Lesotho in the mid-2000s. The Mexico programme formally launched in 2011 after decades of partnership with local groups, and PIH formalized a partnership with the Navajo Nation in 2009, named COPE (Community Outreach and Patient Empowerment). PIH has long supported MDR-TB efforts in former USSR states, most recently in Kazakhstan since 2009. The Ebola epidemic brought PIH to Sierra Leone and Liberia in 2014.

Nature of partnerships: PIH is often asked by government partners to take the lead on training, curriculum development, and delivery, though in many countries this is done hand in hand through very close government relationships. Reporting is regular, continuous, and aims to be bi-directional.

CHW Cadre

Name of CHW cadre: since PIH works across ten countries, with government and community partners, there are multiple different CHW programmes with many different names. The most common are: accompanier, accompagnateur, acompañante, cuidadora, binome, maternal mortality reduction agent, maternal health worker, polyvalent community health agent, community health promoter, treatment supporter, or just community health worker.

Core principles of operation: across PIH, CHW programmes take on different characteristics based on local preferences. All programmes, however, hope to adhere to core principles, including:

- CHWs are paid, with a variety of reimbursement packages ranging from food to full salaries.
- They work in vulnerable communities, mostly rural, within a catchment area of hundreds of thousands of people around 'beacon facilities' (clinical centres of excellence for primary, secondary, and higher levels of care).
- Recruitment, training, and maintenance is largely done by PIH staff, but often in line with government preferences and guidelines.
- CHWs are always from the communities they serve, and demonstrate a pro-social attitude of service.

- How many households they serve depends on their responsibilities, but generally PIH aims for fewer household than what is commonly assigned, as the goal is quality and not only coverage.
- Accreditation is a goal across all countries.

Training Approach

There are a variety of training methods and mechanisms across PIH's ten countries. In general:

- CHWs are trained by PIH staff in partnership with government actors.
- The majority of the training is either in groups, or one on one during supervision meetings.
- The most common technology used during training is work tools (digital health tools) and visualization tools (projected videos, charts, etc.).
- The PIH approach to community health is inspired by the values of 'accompaniment' first, and then will include specific task-based trainings depending on the cadre (i.e. iCCM, maternal health, HIV/TB, household registers, etc.).
- Greater weight is given to service, compassion, and addressing vulnerability, than teaching skills for task shifting.
- Most training curricula will be developed with government partners, seeking feedback from community partners.
- Supervision visits are seen as one of the best opportunities to train based on practical experiences. The goal is to mentor towards greater capacity to use good judgement in the more difficult scenarios.
- CHW leaders regularly give feedback on trainings, and often participate in the development of materials.

Format of Training

The majority of PIH projects start with an initial training (of variable length, ranging from a week to months, depending on the CHW model), which is then followed by regular trainings of 1–3 days at least quarterly to monthly. This could be during group administrative meetings, supervision encounters, or other gatherings.

Mentorship and Enhanced Supervision for Healthcare and Quality Improvement, or MESH-QI, is an approach developed for nurses in Rwanda, that has expanded to other PIH sites such as Malawi. The approach to mentoring CHWs is practically similar and philosophically aligned. More information can be found at: https://www.pih.org/practitioner-resource/mesh-qi-implementation-guide

Training Outcomes

Pre- and post-tests are the most common means to assess the outcomes of training, though they take a variety of formats, from written tests to practicums to direct observations.

Pre- and post-tests are regularly deployed with the goal of CHWs passing certain thresholds before certification. If CHWs do not pass, their training is generally augmented until they pass.

Key Lessons for Success

- Select a wide group of candidates, train them all and then select the first cohort from the highest performers. Others can be on a waitlist that continues to get regular trainings and will be ready to fill vacancies as they arise from common reasons for attrition.
- Focus on building capacity to function on a human level first, instead of focusing on gaining knowledge to pass written exams; performance on a written test usually does not predict performance in the field.
- To maximize equity, do not make literacy a minimum standard for selection. Instead, make efforts to augment gaps in literacy in the most pro-social candidates. There are some skills you can't teach (i.e. compassion and passion for serving the vulnerable).
- The most important lessons the CHWs will learn about their job is how they are treated by colleagues, and how their patients are cared for when in the healthcare system. CHWs can only be as strong as the systems they work within.

Key Challenges

- If initial trainings are extensive (i.e. months to years), then they will be expensive, and attrition will be also quite expensive as CHWs take with them all that training. It is likely best to train a minimum to safely start working and then augment their knowledge regularly and consistently. This also helps to retain CHWs because they will be more regularly engaged.
- There are trade-offs between doing what is expedient and cost saving (i.e. making all tests multiple choice written tests) and what is pedagogically the most effective but time consuming (i.e. verbal evaluations of all CHWs). When in doubt, invest more in better systems.
- Technology can add a lot, but fancy new devices and digital interfaces must still follow good teaching principles.
- Other challenges include: lack of standardized certification of CHWs in many countries, a constant need for refresher trainings due to frequent changes in treatment protocols, lack of, or limited, local and national funding for community health programmes, sometimes a limited capacity to communicate easily with CHWs who live in remote and rural areas.

Additional Resources (to be included as part of online resources)

MESH-QI: https://www.pih.org/practitioner-resource/mesh-qi-implementation-guide
Training paper from programme in Guatemala: Lightfoot, M. & Palazuelos, D. (2016). Evaluating the teaching methods of a community health worker training curriculum in rural Guatemala. *Journal of Family Medicine & Community Health*, 3(6), 1096.
Palazuelos, D., Farmer, P., & Mukherjee, J. (2018). Community health and equity of outcomes: The Partners in Health experience. *Lancet Global Health*, 6, e491–3.

Pivot

http://pivotworks.org/

Organizational Profile

Region of operation: Ifandiana District, Madagascar

Partnership model: PIVOT collaborates with the Ministry of Public Health (Ministère de la Santé Publique (MinSanP) in French) to support the public health system, including community health.

Name given to CHWs: Agent communautaire (AC).

Funders: Conservation, Food and Health Foundation; CRI Foundation; IZUMI Foundation; MJS Foundation; Preston-Werner Ventures; Wagner Foundation.

Pivot's Community Health Worker Programme

Historically, in Madagascar, community health workers (CHWs) have been selected by the community, are trained, and receive monthly group supervision at health centres. They are not paid a salary; instead they receive compensation for their work by selling medications with a mark-up, which generates profit for the AC. Community health services are offered at a community health site or other fixed location (e.g. the AC's home or a village building).

As well as providing expanded support for the ACs still working in five other communes, PIVOT is piloting a two-pronged model of community health in the commune of Ranomafana, in Ifanadiana District. The model includes proactive care (household-based surveillance of sick or malnourished children, suspected tuberculosis cases, and pregnant women) combined with fixed community health sites staffed by ACs where sick patients can seek care as needed—and a new model of community health management.

In the pilot commune, each fokontany (a collection of villages in which 750–2500 people reside) has at least three, and as many as five ACs, depending on population size. At least two ACs travel on a circuit throughout the fokontany to conduct home visits to each household, while one AC provides services at a fixed community health site. These responsibilities rotate between ACs in the fokontany. As a part of this pilot system, PIVOT increased the number of ACs per fokontany; existing ACs were retained in the health system, and new ACs were recruited through an open recruitment process. PIVOT provides financial incentive for new ACs which is equivalent to Madagascar's minimum wage.

ACs are not accredited in Madagascar. Historically, ACs have been elders, predominantly male, selected for their position in the community, and there have been no educational requirements. Indeed, many do not have a secondary education, although most are literate. In the pilot commune, the gender divide of ACs is more equitable and nearly 50% of ACs are women.

Training Approach

Under the pilot project, the initial training is 12 days and is mostly didactic. New ACs are trained on the integrated community case management (iCCM) protocol; screening for malnutrition in children under five; and tuberculosis screening, directly observed therapy, and patient education; as well as proactive care. In these sessions ACs also practice skills needed for diagnosis, classification, treatment, and follow-up. In addition to the initial session, there are ongoing training opportunities including refresher trainings and workshops to teach new skills (e.g. dispensing family planning methods).

Training is conducted in a group setting using a combination of lectures and the opportunity for ACs to practice skills and use tools. Training materials are developed by PIVOT's community health team and incorporate MinSanP materials and information as appropriate.

Supervision

All ACs receive *monthly field-based supervision*, which includes direct observation of care provided by ACs to sick children. The supervisor completes an observation checklist on a tablet to document that the AC checks for danger signs, and completes required steps for diagnosis, classification, treatment, and counselling. The data from the checklist generate metrics on quality of care which allow the supervisor to monitor the performance of the ACs over time. The AC supervisor provides feedback on the quality of care that he/she observed the AC provide and checks the completeness and correctness of the data recorded by the AC on forms and registers. During field-based supervision, the AC has the opportunity to ask questions of the supervisor and is observed providing care, so that the supervisor can identify areas where additional support is needed. A *monthly group supervision* meeting is held at the health centre for all ACs in the commune, at which ACs ask questions, receive brief refresher trainings, and update needed supplies and medications. Health centre meetings are also an opportunity for ACs to submit their monthly activity reports, which are then aggregated for all ACs in the commune and submitted to the district as part of the routine monthly reporting process. During such meetings, health facilities are also able to relay specific requests to ACs regarding cases lost to follow-up.

During periodic review meetings, a PIVOT monitoring and evaluation team member joins the head of the health centre, the AC supervisor, and the AC to review supervision results and provide feedback to the AC. PIVOT provides support for the monthly health centre-based supervision meetings and field-based supervision, including paying the salaries of AC supervisors.

Monitoring and Outcomes

The impact of training on knowledge is assessed using a pre/post-test designed by Madagascar's MinSanP. The results of these tests are shared with district government officials. Supervision data and information on quality of care are shared with MinSanP staff, including health centre managers and the district health office. Periodically, PIVOT and district staff will conduct joint work sessions to review data to identify programme priorities and areas needing support.

Practical Tips for Success

- Consistent, monthly supervision, including field-based supervision is an important component of accompaniment and continuous learning.
- AC supervisors require supervision and support. Supervision is an evolving process which can always be improved, and the AC supervisors need assistance in identifying how to meet evolving demands.

- As the portfolio of services offered by ACs expands, we need to consider if additional ACs need to be hired in order to ensure that all tasks are completed and ACs provide high quality care.
- Preliminary results show that the two-pronged approach—where ACs travel proactively to households and one remains stationary at a fixed community health site—increases overall case management. The innovative model places ACs in the field and ensures constant access to care without reducing health seeking at the community health site.
- Paying community health workers a fair wage, aligned with their work and the amount of time that they spend on providing care, is an important component of professionalizing the cadre.

Key Challenges

- ACs identified by the community are often respected elders with limited formal education. As the job description of the AC evolves to include more tasks and more movement, selection criteria have been refined to allow for recruitment of ACs who can complete the work, but who reflect community values and are seen as trusted providers.
- Geographic barriers (distance, terrain, travel time) inhibit contact between the ACs and the community, community members who travel to access ACs, and AC supervisors with ACs. The proactive care model, where an AC travels on a set circuit among homes, reduces barriers to access, but the travel is challenging for ACs.
- Currently, ACs in one commune receive a monthly financial incentive equivalent to Madagascar's minimum wage and the rest receive a stipend plus additional remuneration for attending supervision meetings. Given the workload, the lack of a formal salary for many ACs limits their motivation to provide high quality work.
- PIVOT is working with partners to implement mobile data collection by ACs. The ability to share data between ACs and with facilities is limited by lack of network coverage in Ifanadiana District.

Index